CHEST PAIN

CHEST
PAIN
When &
When Not to
Worry

Albert J. Miller, M.D.

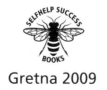

SELFHELP SUCCESS
BOOKS

Gretna 2009

First published by Wellness Institute/Self-Help Books, LLC, 2005
Published by arrangement with the author by
   Selfhelp Success Books, L.L.C., 2009

First printing, 2005
First Selfhelp Success printing, 2009
Second Selfhelp Success printing, 2009

ISBN 9781935235033

Selfhelp Success, Selfhelp Success Books, and
   are imprints of Selfhelp Success Books, L.L.C.

Cover design and artwork by Jason Ladner

Printed in the United States of America
Published by Selfhelp Success Books, L.L.C.
900 Burmaster Street, Gretna, Louisiana 70053

. . . To my wife, my daughter and my patients—
all supportive of my efforts to write this book.

CHEST PAIN
TABLE OF CONTENTS

Introduction

INTRODUCTION————

Chest pain is a common reason for a visit to the cardiologist's office. So I was not surprised when several of my patients, knowing that I had written a book on the **DIAGNOSIS OF CHEST PAIN**, complained, "patients need that kind of book more than doctors!" I tried lending my book to a number of patients, but clearly it was loaded with too much medical jargon to be helpful to them. Having finally decided that patients needed their own book, I found that it was more difficult to write for the lay person than for the physicians. It is not easy to describe pains in a clear and understandable way, and discussing chest pains poses special communication problems.

The main problem for the individual experiencing chest pain is to decide whether the pain is serious and what to do about it. Therefore, the mission of this small book will be to present in understandable language information about the heart and chest pain and to emphasize when to consult a doctor and when to relax. In order to discuss chest pain in a rational manner, I try to present the reader with enough basic medical information to provide an understanding of the origins and mechanisms of chest pain. Although I have tried to accomplish this, the reader should understand that this small book is not meant in any way to replace a skilled physician. On the contrary, it should serve to emphasize the value of the physician's insight.

Who among us has never had a chest pain? Chest

pains are common and though most chest pains are not serious, they almost always produce some anxiety. They often cause concern about heart trouble. Ironically, many significant chest pains are dismissed or ignored as pain because the discomfort is not severe enough to be considered as "a pain." As we shall see, some noteworthy pains do not present in the expected places, and some are quite mild. Most of us have considerable difficulty in describing chest pains, and some may think that this inability is a personal deficiency. It is not a personal deficiency - all of us, including physicians, have difficulty describing chest pains we experience. There are good reasons for this difficulty, and we will explore some of them.

All of us have chest pain at one time or another

Considering that the heart, lungs, diaphragm and chest wall are in constant motion, it is surprising that these structures do not give rise to chest pain more often. Many examples of benign chest pains can be drawn from our everyday lives. One sleeps in a peculiar position and awakens with an aching pain in the left upper chest. Protracted coughing with a cold leads to soreness in the lower chest on both sides. An attack of shingles makes one miserable with a burning chest pain. Abdominal bloating after food indiscretion gives a heavy feeling in the lower chest. The death of a loved one leads to a feeling of weight and oppression on the front of the chest. An inordinately hard sneeze gives a terrible pain on the side of the chest due to a bruised rib.

A miserable burning sensation ("heartburn") under the breastbone in the middle of the chest follows an evening of hot chili and too much beer. And then there are the chest muscle aches and pains that all of us experience, for example, after a day of unaccustomed gardening. Readers can undoubtedly add examples of their own. Obviously, there are many chest pains that are not serious, are not life threatening, and do not require immediate medical attention. And then there are the other kinds of pains - those that should lead one to prompt medical attention. We will discuss the benign and more serious chest pains in some detail.

To present the information in an orderly and understandable manner, I have categorized the various kinds of pains based on their anatomical origin. The first three chapters discuss aspects of the history of our knowledge of chest pain, the anatomy of the chest organs, and the nature of pain. Hopefully this background will provide the reader with enough information to make the subsequent chapters more interesting and understandable. Not every kind of pain is discussed, but rather emphasis is put on illustrating those pains that should lead us to medical care and those pains that need not worry us.

CHAPTER I

THE HISTORY |
—— of our knowledge of
CHEST PAIN |

It is amazing how little information is available about chest pain from the writings of antiquity, and those brief mentions of chest pain that we have are vague and lack detail. In the 1500s, Vesalius wrote about "a sad feeling and pain in the heart." Around that time the Florentine physician Benivieni described a woman who was sometimes troubled with "pain at her heart." He stated, "At last the pain began to attack her more frequently and at length she was carried off." A gentleman who was not a physician, Edward, Earl of Clarendon (1609-1674), probably wrote the first meaningful description of pain originating from heart disease when he described his father's illness. "He was seized by so sharp a pain in the left arm...that the torment made him pale as he was dead; and he used to say that he had passed the pangs of death and that he should die with one of these fits; as soon as it was over, which was quickly, he was the cheerfullest man living."

1

In 1649 the great physician William Harvey described a patient who "made complaint of a certain distressing pain in the chest, especially in the night season; so that dreading at one time syncope, at another suffocation in his attacks he led an unquiet and anxious life."

But it was left to William Heberden, (**Figure 1**) an astute British physician, to open the door to our study of chest pain when he provided in 1772 the first succinct account of a pain originating from the heart that he called "angina pectoris." Heberden wrote,

"There is a disorder of the breast, marked with strong and peculiar symptoms, considerable for the kind of danger

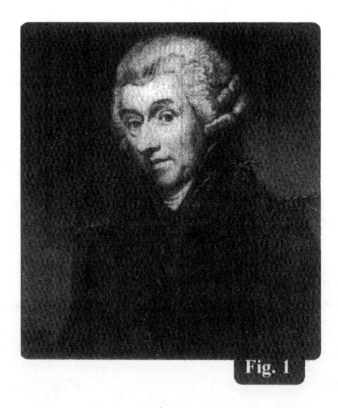

Fig. 1

belonging to it, and not extremely rare, of which I do not recollect any mention among medical authors. The seat of it, and sense of strangling and anxiety with which it is attended, may make it not improperly called Angina pectoris."

"Those, who are afflicted with it, are seized, while they are walking, and more particularly when they walk soon after eating, with a painful and most disagreeable sensation in the breast, which seems as if it would take their life away, if it were to increase or continue: the moment they stand still, all this uneasiness vanishes. In all other respects the patients are at the beginning of this disorder perfectly well, and in particular have no shortness of breath, from which it is totally different."

The fact is that Heberden did not know the cause of the pain that he so well described. It remained for others to relate angina pectoris to heart disease and it is likely that Edward Jenner, the originator of the vaccination against smallpox, did understand the relationship between angina pectoris and disease of the coronary arteries. Jenner's good friend, John Hunter, himself a physician who was honored as the father of surgery, had angina pectoris. From Jenner's letters it would appear that he correctly related angina pectoris to coronary artery disease, but he apparently refrained from publishing his observations to avoid causing Hunter undue emotional distress. Hunter did ultimately die from his heart disease.

Almost 150 years passed before the description of

an acute myocardial infarction (commonly known as a "heart attack") was first published by Obrastzow and Straschesko in Russia in 1910 and soon afterwards in the United States by Herrick, in 1912. These publications about the diagnosis of a heart attack ("myocardial infarction") were particularly important because they showed for the first time that the diagnosis of this serious heart condition could be made in living patients. Prior to that time various chest pains were related to diseases of the heart, but these diseases were considered uniformly fatal. These important publications did not have an immediate impact, but gradually physicians began to make the diagnosis of coronary artery disease in living patients, and the field blossomed when various medical interventions made it possible to do something positive for heart attack patients.

Descriptions and understanding of chest pains other than those from the heart are surprisingly recent. The pain associated with disease of the lower esophagus (the swallowing tube that passes from the throat to the stomach) was first appreciated in the early 1900s, and inflammation of the lower esophagus as a source of pain was first described as recently as 1935. The term "reflux esophagitis" was proposed as recently as 1951. Pains of skeletal origin, including pain from the vertebrae (bones forming the spinal column) in the neck, required the perfection of x-ray techniques. As recently as 1936 there was little information available on pain arising from disease of the spine in the neck. In more recent times the diagnosis of skeletal abnormalities has become very sophisticated because of advances in radiological and other imaging methods.

Understandably, physicians became more interested in chest pains as they became able to do something about the pathology that caused them. And certainly our ability to deal with chest pains of a serious nature, such as those from the heart, has increased strikingly since the time of World War II. Indeed, it is the heart that remains the main focus of attention to chest pain to this day. That is not surprising considering that there is so very much to do to help patients with acute or chronic heart disease. Our knowledge about heart disease and our ability to treat it is due to a great extent to the remarkable achievements of the biomedical engineers, physicists, chemists and pharmacologists.

CHAPTER II

ANATOMY
of the
CHEST

If you ask most people to point to their heart, they point to the left side of the chest. Indeed, patients come to see me, point to the left side of the chest near or to the left of the nipple, and say "I have a pain in my heart." Actually, the heart is in the middle of the chest, leaning somewhat more to the left than the right. **Figure 2** shows the heart as you would "see" it looking at the front of another individual (or as a doctor "sees" it looking at a patient sitting in front of him). The lungs surround the heart at each side. The trachea ("the windpipe"), which you can feel in front of the neck as a rounded tube, carries air from the nasal passages and the back of the throat to the bronchi, which are the large tubes going to the lungs. The bronchi divide into smaller channels, the bronchioles. The bronchioles pass to the thin-walled alveoli sacs, where oxygen is taken up and carbon dioxide is released. The heart "sits" on the diaphragm below. The diaphragm is the muscular organ that separates the chest from the

6

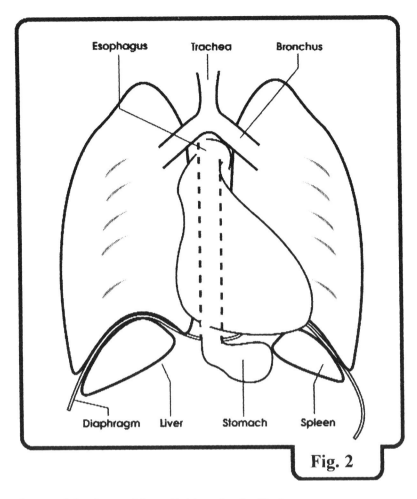

Organs of the chest and immediately under the diaphram.

abdomen. It is important in the mechanics of breathing. Poliomyelitis ("polio") is one of the diseases that can injure the nerve control of the diaphragm and lead to marked breathing problems.

Note how close the organs are to each other. The stomach resides under the left side of the diaphragm, and

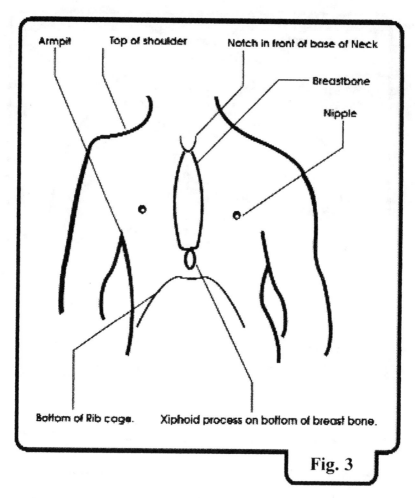

Armpit   Top of shoulder   Notch in front of base of Neck

Breastbone

Nipple

Bottom of Rib cage.   Xiphoid process on bottom of breast bone.

Fig. 3

Showing major landmarks that are useful in describing chest pain.

to its left is the spleen.   Under the right side of the
diaphragm is the liver.   If you poke a finger under your
right lowest rib you will be aiming towards the gall
bladder, which is nestled under the liver. The esophagus
("swallowing tube") is just behind the heart; in fact, the
heart often normally leans against it. Before the days of
modern imaging techniques we would use fluoroscopy to

visualize the heart. By having the patient swallow barium during the examination we were aided in evaluating the size and shape of one of the heart chambers. The esophagus carries swallowed food down to the stomach by passing through an opening in the diaphragm. Sometimes this opening is too large and will allow part or all of the stomach to pass up into the chest, a so-called hiatal hernia.

We can think of the chest as a big barrel covered with muscle and skin, extending from the neck on top to the bottom of the rib cage below. There are various places on the surface of the chest that are useful landmarks to the physician and are helpful in localizing pains. An observant patient can relate pain or discomfort to these landmarks, and thus can be very helpful to the doctor. **Figure 3** illustrates the landmarks that are easy to identify. These landmarks frequently are used in writing and in discussion by physicians. Some examples include:

Notch in front of neck	**suprasternal notch**
Breastbone	**sternum**
Lowest part of breastbone	**xiphoid process**
Armpit	**axilla**
Bottom of rib cage	**lower costal margin**
Where the boney part of the rib meets the cartilage part	**costochondral junction**
Where the rib attaches to the breastbone	**costosternal junction**

9

In the chest wall, beneath the skin, are the ribs, the muscles between them, and the big muscles on top of them. Under the skin, and also between the ribs, are arteries, veins, nerves, lymphatics, fat, and connective tissues.

The inside lining of the chest is a thin, smooth, glistening layer called the pleura, which also covers the chest cavity side of the diaphragm and the lungs themselves. As the lungs expand and deflate, their surfaces glide smoothly over the pleura on the inside of the chest wall. The heart also has a thin smooth layer on its surface and sits in a sac lined with a glistening membrane, the pericardial sac. A little fluid is always present in the pericardial sac, so the heart normally contracts in a sac with a nicely lubricated inner surface.

The main pumping chamber of the heart is the left ventricle, which pumps blood out a large artery, the aorta, and on throughout the body. Arising from the right ventricle of the heart is the pulmonary artery, which pumps blood to the lungs to receive oxygen. **Figure 4** is a diagram of the heart and the major blood vessels. The blood that has received oxygen in the lungs passes back to the heart in the pulmonary veins. The pulmonary veins empty into an antechamber, the left atrium. From the left atrium the blood passes to the left ventricle to be pumped to the body. Blood from the body, where much of its oxygen and nutrients has been removed, returns to an antechamber, the right atrium, via large veins known as the superior and inferior vena cavae. From the right

10

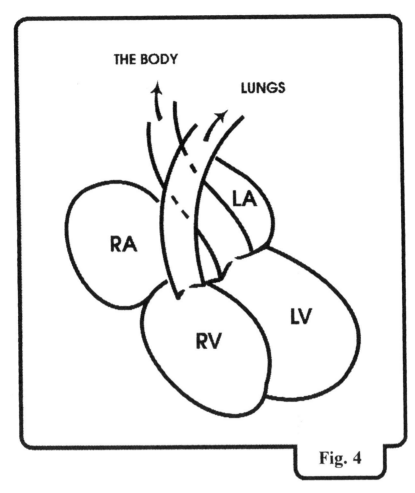

THE BODY

LUNGS

RA

LA

LV

RV

Fig. 4

The four chambers of the heart and the main vessels leaving the right and left ventricles. The blood from the body comes back to the right atrium, passes to the right ventricle (RV) and is then pumped through the pulmonary artery to the lungs. The oxygenated blood comes back to the left atrium, passes to the left ventricle (LV) and is then pumped out the aorta to the body.

atrium blood passes to the right ventricle, which pumps it to the lungs again to be oxygenated.

It is remarkable and noteworthy that the diaphragm, the

11

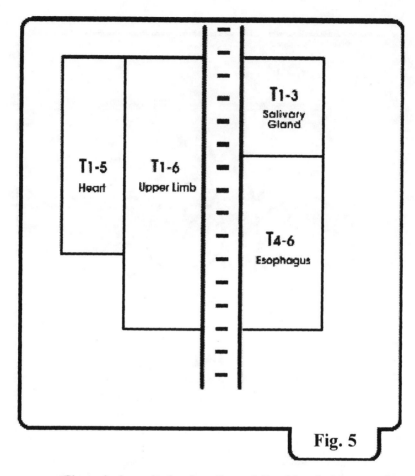

Fig. 5

The spinal cord showing the relationships between various sympathetic nervous system connector cells. Note that the heart, upper limbs and esophagus overlap each other.

muscles of the chest wall, the lungs and the heart are in constant motion from the time of our birth to our death.

All of the organs of the chest have arteries, veins and nerves. Some of them share nerves originating from common sites. Thus, for example, the heart, the lower portion of the

12

esophagus and the upper limbs have overlapping nerve connections to the spinal cord (**Figure 5**). It is important for the physician to understand these concepts in order to reach a correct diagnosis of chest pain. The overlapping nerve supply to organs is one of the body characteristics that make determining the origin of a chest pain so difficult at times.

Two important anatomical aspects of the organs of the chest that relate to chest pain should be stressed:

● The organs of the chest and those under the diaphragm are intimately close to each other and often share nerve supplies. There are no empty spaces between the organs of the chest.

● Chest pain may arise from any of the many organs and structures that comprise the chest wall, and from the organs within, above and beneath the chest cavity.

CHAPTER III

THE NATURE of CHEST PAIN

Somatic and visceral pains

Definitions:

"**Visceral**" -referring to the large organs in any one of the body cavities.

"**Somatic**" - pertaining to the body wall rather than the viscera.

For our discussion purposes, there are two types of pain: "somatic" and "visceral". I have modified the technical definitions somewhat to make them more understandable. *Somatic* pains are relatively easy to localize and describe. If you are stuck in the skin of the arm with a sharp needle, even if your eyes are closed, you can immediately localize the pain and describe it as sharp. A cut on the skin is promptly localized and identified. If you bump your elbow, you know right away where it hurts. If a person breaks a rib in a fall, the area of pain is recognized and the circumstances that make it worse, such as pressing on the rib or a deep breath or a cough, are readily apparent. These are somatic pains, and the discomfort that is experienced is localized to the site of the injury or pathology. Our brains learn to identify pains and their origins on our body surfaces, broadly speaking, with a high degree of accuracy. We respond to this information promptly and most often appropriately. A bleeding painful cut on a finger, for example, is immediately treated with pressure to stop the bleeding and bandaging. These body surface signals protect us by helping us to survive in an external environment. But it is a totally different story when we deal with visceral pain.

Pains of visceral origin arise from the organs within or beneath the chest and are difficult to describe and difficult to localize. They tend to be vague, diffuse in nature, and the pain they cause is usually felt on the surface of the body. In other words, the pain is referred to a surface area from an inner organ of origin. One possible explanation for referred pain was offered by MacKenzie in 1923 (**Figures 6a-b**). Pain originating from the heart is referred pain. Thus, we don't feel pain from the heart within the heart itself, but rather we feel pain, for example, behind the breastbone in the middle of the chest. Pain from internal organs, the viscera, can be referred to surfaces of the body quite distant from the organ itself. Thus, pain due to insufficient blood to a portion of the

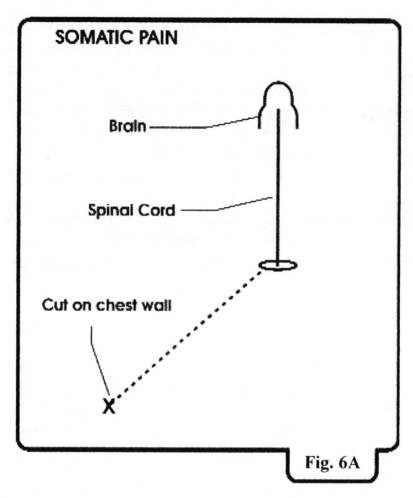

SOMATIC PAIN

Brain

Spinal Cord

Cut on chest wall

X

Fig. 6A

The pain impulse travels from a cut of the skin to the spinal cord and up to
the brain, where it is properly interpreted and located.

heart can be felt as pain in the left shoulder. In
medical jargon, an inadequate supply of blood to an
organ is termed "ischemia" of the tissue involved.
Ischemia of a part of the heart muscle that occurs
during fast walking can cause an aching pain in the
left forearm that is relieved by resting.

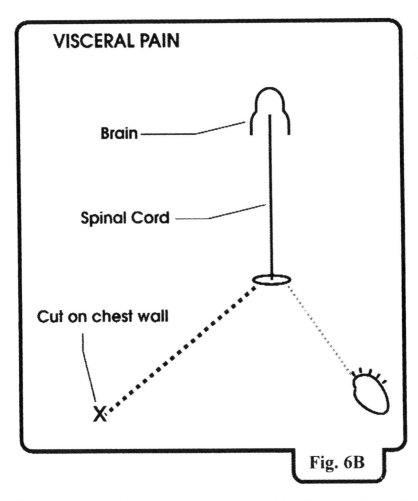

VISCERAL PAIN

Brain

Spinal Cord

Cut on chest wall

X

Fig. 6B

The pain impulse originates in the heart muscle and travels to the spinal cord. When the impulse reaches the brain, it is interpreted as coming from point X. Thus, the pain is "referred."

We will deal with somatic and referred visceral pains in more detail when we discuss pain arising from specific organs. But for now, it should be understood that describing visceral referred pains is always difficult, even for nurses and doctors who are trained in using medical terminology.

17

The descriptive language of chest pains

The words used to describe chest pain

Patients have a tough time finding words to describe pains arising from the heart and the other organs related to the chest. Keep in mind that we are using a broad definition of "pain" that includes such experiences as mild discomfort. It is important to stress this point because often no correlation exists between the severity of a pain and the extent of disease it reflects. As we have mentioned, and will continue to stress, there is, for example, no correlation between the severity of angina pectoris (caused by a decrease in blood supply to a part of the heart muscle; "ischemia" of the heart muscle) and the extent of the coronary artery disease (atherosclerosis; "hardening of the arteries") that causes it. A feeling of mild tightness behind the breastbone on exertion can reflect severe coronary atherosclerosis involving all three major branches.

When seeking the words to describe chest pain, patients often start off describing what it does not feel like. "It isn't really a pain." "I don't know how to describe it. It's not sharp and it doesn't last very long." "It's really not very uncomfortable." But then, often after some prodding from the doctor, words are

18

Descriptive Words for Chest Pain.

-Dull	-Grabbing
-Aching Pressing	-Piercing
-Constricting	-Throbbing
-Heavy	-Pounding
-Weight on my chest	-Shooting
-Squeezing	-Boring
-Expanding	-Gnawing
-Sharp	-Cramping
-Knifelike	-Crushing
-Cutting	-Pulling
-Burning	-Tingling
-Searing	-Stinging
-Sticking	-Tearing
-Catching	-Penetrating
-Pinching	-Twisting a Knot

Table-1

used to try to describe what the pain feels like. Some of those words are listed in **Table 1**. Not all of the words refer to pain of a serious nature. Indeed, some of them immediately point to a benign origin of the pain.

Patients often insist that their chest discomfort is not a "pain" per se. The conversation often goes something like this:

> "Well, Mrs. Jones, tell me about your chest pain."
> "But, doctor, I don't have chest pain."
> "Do you have any chest discomfort?"
> "Yes, I do. I get this mild tightness in the front of my chest and in the throat when I'm walking fast, particularly when I'm rushing. <u>But it isn't a pain</u>, and it goes away as soon as I slow down."

Though Mrs. Jones denies having "pain," the tightness that she describes is considered a form of pain by physicians. She doesn't categorize it as a pain because it is not very severe, but nevertheless, it can have considerable medical significance.

The severity of pain

Patients tend to deal with pain on the basis of its severity, and this proclivity often becomes a major problem in communicating with doctors. The patient is asked whether he or she has chest pain, and as noted in the example above, the answer is "No, I have no pain at all." Then, on further questioning, "But I do get this tightness in the middle of the chest when I walk fast. It's quite mild and isn't really a pain." The opposite circumstance with a chest pain may be seen when a young anxious woman patient describes "a terrible, sharp pain under the left breast." The pain comes and goes, and taking a deep breath is a misery

20

because it makes the pain worse. "I have to take shallow breaths until finally, after about five minutes, the pain goes away." In this instance the patient describes a rather severe pain that is not of serious significance except that it is frightening, which I have named a "precordial catch." I published a couple of papers on this subject, mainly to emphasize that it is a completely benign pain, though I admit that we still do not know its cause. Most patients consider "pain" to be a particularly severe discomfort, and it is also dependant on individual thresholds for pain (**Figure 7**). A toothache is a pain. A twisted ankle that is swollen and every step a misery is an ankle pain. A severe sharp shooting lancinating pain in the scalp is a pain.

We all have had chest pains that have nothing to do with the heart. A good example is the misnamed "heartburn," a mid chest burning pain that is often associated with reflux of acid stomach contents into the lower esophagus.

I have presented examples to show that the severity of a pain may not be related to its seriousness. This truism applies to angina pectoris (insufficient blood to the heart muscle as, for example, with exercise), but does not apply to heart attacks ("myocardial infarction"). Some severe pains are very serious. Severe pain in the middle of the chest may indicate a heart attack or an impending heart attack and calls for an emergency response.

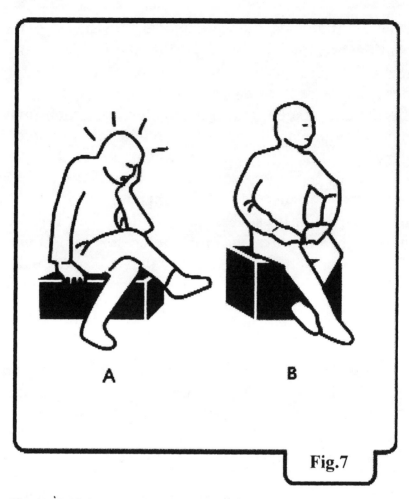

A   B

Fig.7

The threshold for pain varies form person to person. On a scale of 1 to 10, where 10 is the worst, patient A rates the pain at 10 and the patient B rates it at 2.

It is apparent that one cannot determine the seriousness of a particular chest pain by its severity alone. Mild pains can be serious and more severe pains may be benign. As noted before, an accurate description of what the pain feels like can be helpful in determining its significance.

The duration of pain

The duration of a pain is an important clue to its origin and seriousness. Transitory pains lasting just a few seconds, including sharp shooting pains, are rarely of any significance. The sharp shooting scalp pain is an example. We all get them. Chest pains that persist for many hours and days and that are aggravated by movement of some kind, like reaching for the coffee pot or putting things on a high shelf, are invariably musculoskeletal in origin. They merit attention, but not as an emergency. In contrast, a heaviness or tightness in the middle of the chest precipitated by physical exertion or emotional stress, lasting a few to ten minutes, and relieved by rest is likely angina pectoris, a pain originating from the heart, and should not be ignored. A pain in the middle of the chest that is persistent, whether it is severe or less severe, merits attention. A pain on either side of the chest that stays and is aggravated by taking a deep breath, whether it is severe or not so severe, calls for medical attention even though it is not from the heart. Realistically, severe pains, persistent or recurrent, irrespective of location, should lead one to seek medical attention. Even if a pain is not of a serious nature, its persistence is disturbing and it should be alleviated if possible.

Pain actually is a friend to the sufferer in that it calls for action. The person who has pain with a heart attack and promptly seeks medical attention is much better off than the person who has little discomfort and procrastinates about dealing with it. But some persons who get an adequate warning of trouble still procrastinate.

Recently a patient of ours, a 67 year old man being treated for high blood pressure, phoned one of my partners in the evening to report a pain that he described as coming from his "hiatal hernia." The pain, in the lower part of the middle of the chest, had been present for about 2 hours. My partner was concerned about the possibility the pain might be coming from the heart and urged the patient to go immediately to a close by hospital emergency room. Because the pain was only moderate in intensity the patient decided to wait, and finally went to the emergency room some 3 hours later only at his wife's insistence. He had had a massive myocardial infarction ("heart attack") and developed congestive heart failure. Some days later, after treatment had stabilized his medical condition, he had coronary bypass surgery. After surgery he had a stormy postoperative recovery, but went home after about 10 days in the hospital. He is feeling better now, but his procrastination early in his illness caused him to lose a significant portion of his left ventricular heart muscle, a loss that he will have to deal with for the rest of his life.

The location of pain

Pain nerves to the chest wall arise from the spinal cord in the neck and upper back, which is protected by the spine (the vertebral column). There is an important concept that merits emphasis here - pain is felt at the point where a nerve serves the tissue or organ, and not at the origin of the nerve. Thus, as we will discuss more, irritation of nerves in the neck by arthritis can cause pain to be felt in the front of the upper chest.

The location of a pain is important, and provides information about its origin. Pain in the middle of the chest suggests the heart or esophagus. Pain in the pit of the stomach is usually from the stomach or first part of the intestine, but may be from the heart or lower esophagus. Pains on the sides of the chest are usually from the chest wall or the lungs. Pain on the top of the left shoulder may come from the heart, the lining around the heart or the left side of the diaphragm, being a particular kind of referred pain. Pain in the left upper arm can be from the heart, shoulder or neck. Pain in the neck, the jaw or the throat can be from the heart, or from a local problem. The location of the pain helps in determining its origin, but it can be misleading to the uninitiated. The potential for confusion and understandable procrastination about some pains related to disease of chest organs results from the way the pain is referred (**Figure 8**). Thus, for example, pain from the heart can be felt solely in the left shoulder area, or in the jaw, or in the throat. Because the location of the pain can be confusing, the information provided about precipitating circumstances is particularly important. A pain in the left jaw when chewing food or drinking cold liquids is likely from a problem with a tooth. However, a pain in the left jaw precipitated by walking after the evening meal and relieved by rest is likely from the heart.

Mr. S.J., a 45-year old lawyer, saw his dentist because of recurrent pain in his left lower jaw. The pain was not severe, but was quite bothersome, and occurred particularly after eating. The dentist found no local problem, but elicited the history that Mr. J. would take a walk after his evening meal, and the pain was most likely to occur during that walk. We saw the patient on referral from the dentist, and confirmed the circumstances of when the jaw pain occurred. The pain was reproduced during a treadmill exercise test and was associated with marked abnormalities in the electrocardiogram. Coronary angiography revealed a 90 percent narrowing in the left circumflex coronary artery. After angioplasty and stenting of the narrowed area the patient had no further jaw pain with walking.

As has been stressed before, persistent or recurrent pain, irrespective of its location, calls for medical attention.

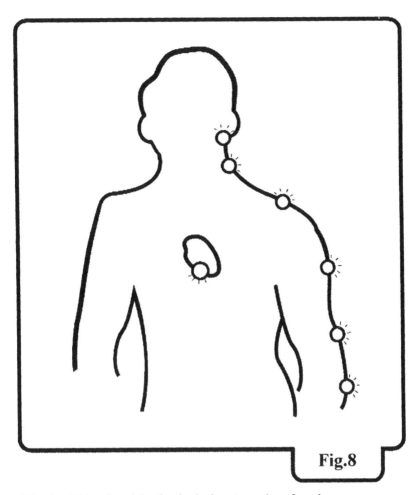

Fig.8

Sites to which pain originating in the heart may be referred.

What brings on the pain, what company does it keep and what relieves it

A burning pain in the middle of the chest that occurs one hour after eating a bowl of hot chili and is eased by chewing an antacid is most likely due to irritation of the lower esophagus from regurgitated acid secretions from the stomach ("reflux"). The usual term used to describe such a pain is "heartburn," but this has absolutely nothing to do with the heart. A burning pain in the middle of the chest that occurs in the morning when getting ready to go to work, that persists and is associated with feeling rather faint and anxious may well be from the heart. A tightness in the throat that occurs when walking in a cold wind and is relieved by going into a warm building and resting for a few minutes is likely from the heart. A pain in the front of the chest and on the top of the left shoulder that occurs a few days after a cold and bronchitis and that is eased by leaning forward may be from a virus inflammation of the sac around the heart. A sharp severe pain on the side of the chest that comes on suddenly three days after a long plane trip and that is made worse by a deep breath or cough may be a blood clot to the lung that has traveled from the leg. We will discuss specific examples later, but suffice it to say here that the symptoms and circumstances that accompany a pain are important in defining its origin, and what relieves the pain is also important. **Table 2** is a questionnaire that our practice group used in doing a research study. As you can see, considerable information can be obtained about any particular chest pain.

Table-2.

Questionnaire Used In the Study of Chest Pain

Name:_____ Age:____ Sex:____ Race:_____

Body build: thin___ Normal___ Stocky___ Obese___ Big-chested___   Date:_____

Concerning the Chest Pain:

WHERE ORIGINATED?

___Retrosternal, high
___Retrosternal, mid
___Retrosternal, low
___Parasternal Lt
___Parasternal Rt
___Mid Lt chest
___Lower Lt Chest
___Upper Lt Chest
___Mid Rt Chest

___Lower Rt Chest
___Upper Rt Chest
___Epigastrium
___Xiphoid Process
___Unbilicus
___Lt Shoulder
___Lt Upper Arm
___Lt Forearm
___Lt Wrist

___Lt Axilla
___Under Lt Shoulder Blade
___Rt Shoulder
___Rt Upper Arm
___Tr Forearm
___Rt Wrist
___Rt Neck
___Lt Neck
___Bilat Neck

___Lt Face
___Rt Face
___Interscapular
Other_____
_____
_____

CHARACTER:

___Dull
___Aching
___Pressing
___Constricting
___Heavy
___Weight on my chest
___Squeezing
___Expanding

___Sharp
___Knifelike
___Cutting
___Burning
___Searing
___Slicking
___Catching
___Pinching

___Grabbing
___Piercing
___Throbbing
___Pounding
___Shooting
___Boring
___Gnawing
___Cramping

___Crushing
___Pulling
___Tingling
___Tearing
___Penetrating
___Other:_____
_____
_____

Variability in character of pain

___Lasts longer from one time to another
___Severity varies
___Radiates when more severe

___Radiation less when pain more severe
___Variable site of onset of pain

Radiation:

___Up retrosternal
___Down retrosternal
___Upper Lt chest
___Mid LT chest
___Low Lt chest
___Under LT Breast
___LT axilla
___Lt neck

___Lt face
___Lt jaw
___Rt teeth
___Lt teeth
___Throat
___Epigastrium
___Rt neck
___Upper Rt chest

___Mid Rt chest
___Low Rt chest
___Lt shoulder
___Lt Upper arm
___Lt forearm
___Lt wrist
___Rt shoulder
___Rt upper arm

___Rt forearm
___Rt wrist
___Interscapular area
___Under Lt shoulder
___Under Rt shoulder
___Both shoulders
___Other:_____
_____

Skin Sensations:

___Tingling
___Crawling
___Burning

___Soreness
___Sensitive
___Tender

___Peculiar
___Numbness
___Feels funny to touch

___Pins & needles
___Other:_____
_____

Duration:

___Seconds
___Transitory
___Like snap of fingers
___1-2 minutes
___3-5 minutes
___5-10 minutes

___10-20 minutes
___20-30 minutes
___30-60minutes
___Hours
___All day
___More than 1 day

___Comes & goes
___When it comes, lasts for days
___Wanes and wanes, but never gone
___Variable, from minutes to hours
___Other_____

Precipitating factors for pain

___Rushing
___Hurrying
___Feeling of being late
___Emotional stress
___Anger
___Joy
___Anxiety

___When scared
___Lifting
___Reaching up
___Making a bed
___Vacuuming
___Tennis
___Walking

___Walking up hill
___Walking in cold
___Cold wind
___Intercourse
___Walking up 1 flight stairs
___Walking up 2 flight stairs
___Dreams

___Eating
___Walking after eating
___Occurs at rest
___Occurs when lying down
___Awakened with pain
___Other:_____

Relief of pain:

__With rest	down	__Change thoughts	__Salve
__Subl ntg	__Antacids	__Relaxing	__Slowing down
__Walking	__Belching	__Aspirin	__Cab blockers
__Standing	__Eating something	__Tylenol	__Beta blockers
__Sitting	__Milk	__Pain medicine	__Nitrates
__Lying down	__Laxative	__Pressing on sore spot	__Narcotics
__Change of posture	__Bowel movement	__Heat application	__Other:_____
__Coughing	__Hot Water	__Cold application	
__Straining or bearing	__Enema	__Massage	

Symptoms in addition to pain:

__Shortness of breath	__Cough	__Gas	__Hiccups
__Palpitations	__Heartburn	__Cramps	__Belch
__Fear	__Dizziness	__Soreness	__Trouble getting enough
__Anxiety	__Faintness	__Aching	air in lungs
__Heart skips beats	__Weakness of areas	__Swelling	__Other:_____
__Heart flip/flops	__Overall Weakness	__Bloating	

Procedures:

_____
_____
_____
_____

Diagnosis:

_____
_____
_____
_____

Chest pain and gender

Physicians have become appropriately aware of the fact that women experience coronary heart disease, even in the pre-menopausal years. This insight is relatively recent, inasmuch as for many years physicians have been taught that menstruating women do not have coronary heart disease and do not suffer "heart attacks," and that women became susceptible to atherosclerosis only when they entered the menopause.

It is only recently that this misinformation has been dispelled. In my experience women have chest pains, as well as the other kinds of pains from coronary heart disease, just as do men. At times these pains are atypical, as they also are in men. In the past women were told that as long as they were menstruating they were protected, and understandably many of them ignored their own discomforts and focused their worry on their male companions and relatives.

Now that we are fully aware of the fact that menstruating women get coronary heart disease before and after menopause, it is important that women pay as much attention to their bodily pains as should men. Indeed, women, who usually have closer relationships with physicians than do men, should insist that their pains and discomforts be given as much attention as is given to their male counterparts.

CHAPTER IV

CHEST PAINS

&

EMOTIONAL STRESS

Emotional stress is a potent stimulator of angina pectoris, the term for the pain from the heart due to decreased blood supply to some portion of it. Indeed, sometimes patients will report chest tightness, heaviness or squeezing pain with emotional stress and not with physical stress.

Mrs. R.R., a 41-year old management consultant, was having marital difficulties. Lately, she and her husband had been arguing about his unwillingness to help around the house, their 12-year old daughter's friends and his tenuous job situation. For about 6 weeks she had noted that these arguments were often associated with an uncomfortable pressure in front of the chest that tended to radiate up towards the neck. The pressure made her anxious, and she would feel better when she walked into another room and relaxed a bit. A treadmill exercise test with rather limited exercise was unremarkable. Nevertheless, diagnostic coronary angiography was recommended and accomplished. The coronary arteries had only moderate atherosclerotic disease not requiring balloon angioplasty or surgery, but in one of the vessels there was observed definite spasm (a constriction due to inappropriate contraction of muscles in the wall of the coronary artery) that was relieved with nitroglycerine. At the time that this spasm was observed Mrs. R. reported that she was having the same kind of chest pain that had been occurring with emotional stress. She felt fine and had no more chest pain after being put on medication for her heart problem, medication that prevented the spasm of the coronary arteries. She was also of the opinion that a divorce from an unpleasant marital situation helped.

On occasion we see a patient who has spasm (constriction) of a coronary artery causing a decreased blood flow to a portion of the heart muscle with emotional stress, perhaps also with physical stress, and no discernible disease of the coronary arteries. However, most frequently, spasm of the muscle in an area of a coronary artery is associated with local disease, almost always atherosclerosis. Obviously, the treatment is to prevent the coronary artery spasm with medications that relax the muscular wall in the coronary artery. A nitroglycerine tablet under the tongue usually is effective in relaxing the muscular coronary artery once the pain has occurred, and at times this medication can be used to prevent the pain.

Emotional stress throws a load on the heart. Certain hormones, for example, adrenalin (epinephrine), are released, the blood pressure may go up, the heart rate increases, the force of heart muscle contraction is increased, and so on. The increase in sympathetic nervous system activity and pouring out of certain hormones from the adrenal gland has been termed "the flight or fight" reaction. In other words, the body gets "keyed up" to fight or run away from danger. Certain athletes, for example, sprint runners, may have such reactions before the starting gun is fired. These reactions, not necessarily undesirable in many life situations, understandably throw an added workload on the heart.

Patients often present themselves to the doctor with a story of recurrent sharp pain on the left side of the chest that causes them considerable anxiety.

Mrs. L.Z., a 34-year old tall thin woman, an accountant and homemaker, came to see me and expressed considerable anxiety about her heart. "Doctor, for about six weeks I have been getting severe heart pains." "Tell me, Mrs. Z.," I asked, "What do you mean by 'heart pains'?" "Well, I know they are pains from my heart because they hit me right under my left breast, where the heart is." The pains that she then described were sharp, rather severe, knife-like and transitory in nature. "They last as long as the snap of my fingers and come at odd times, but they worry me so!" "You know, my mother died of heart trouble when she was 55 years old, and here I am having heart trouble at a much younger age."

Mrs. Z. did not have heart trouble. I explained to her that the heart is not under her left breast and that the pains she was having were not from the heart. Such pains are invariably musculoskeletal in origin and are of no serious significance. Because of her family history, we did an electrocardiogram, checked her cholesterol pattern and did a treadmill exercise test. Everything turned out quite normal and we referred her back to her internist, who later informed us that her pains had disappeared.

Patients always ask whether their coronary artery disease could have been produced by emotional stress. The patient at the beginning of this chapter felt that her heart problem was caused by her marital difficulties. We have no clear evidence supporting the concept that emotional stress is a factor in producing coronary atherosclerosis, though some physicians do believe that chronic severe emotional stress is a risk factor contributing to the production of coronary atherosclerosis. It has been emphasized by some cardiologists that so-called type A personalities, persons who are with high energy, ambitious, driving, time-oriented, are more likely to get heart attacks. On the other hand, some studies show that patients with emotional depression do less well than such type A persons after experiencing a heart attack. We know that severe emotional or physical stress can precipitate a heart attack (myocardial infarction) in persons with preexisting coronary artery disease, and as I have stressed, emotional stress is a potent stimulus for anginal pain. Patients with chronic stable angina pectoris (due to coronary atherosclerosis) learn to avoid those kinds of emotional and physical stress that precipitate their pain. Examples of such adaptations would include changing one's stride to walk somewhat more slowly, changing golf partners to less contentious ones, avoiding confrontations with a teenage son who is going through a rebellious phase, letting your partner at work discipline an errant employee, and learning not to over-react to an excessively nagging boss. However, sometimes patients don't want to adapt their lifestyles to the realities of their being, as the example to follow demonstrates.

Mr. T. R., a 41-year old master plumber, informed me that he enjoyed life and wasn't going to monkey around with all the "don'ts" in the world. When seen in our office for an examination related to an insurance application he reported that his father and uncle had died of heart attacks in their early 50s. His mother had diabetes, but did not require insulin. He was smoking $1^{1/2}$ packs of cigarettes daily and averaged two six-packs of beer a week. On physical examination his height was 5 feet 10 inches, and he was manifestly overweight at 215 pounds. His blood pressure was mildly elevated at 160/95 mm Hg. His cholesterol was elevated to 260 mg and the good fraction, the HDL, was on the low side at 32 mg. He was advised to lose weight, get treatment for his blood pressure and elevated blood cholesterol and cautioned to do a better job in his personal health habits.

It was clear that Mr. R. was quite unimpressed with the advice. About 2 years later we were informed that he had died suddenly when at a football game. His sister told us that he was standing and shouting about a bad play execution on the part of the home team quarterback when he suddenly collapsed. Attempts to resuscitate him were unsuccessful.

Patients bring varying attitudes towards the news that they have a heart problem. Sometimes anxieties about diagnostic tests and treatment approaches have deleterious effects on patients with heart disease. In 1628, the famous physician, William Harvey, wrote "Every affection of the mind that is attended with either pain or pleasure, hope or fear, is the cause of an agitation whose influence extends to the heart." The following patient example illustrates how marked anxiety can influence health care.

Mr. C.C., a PhD in chemistry, a scholar on the editorial boards of a number of journals, the chief of a major biochemistry department, an author of many erudite scientific papers, came to see me with a classic story of increasing angina of effort. His angina had started about 2 years previous, when he was age 55 years, and had gradually been worsening. It reached the point where he got angina, experienced as a disturbing tightness in the middle of his chest, with walking only five or six blocks. Walking during cold weather or in a wind was even worse. Nitroglycerine tablets under the tongue and resting relieved the pain. I advised various tests to assess the status of his coronary artery circulation, and he refused all of them. "Doctor," said he, "I want no tests and refuse to have any kind of treatment interventions such as angioplasty or surgery, and just want you to treat me medically to the best of your ability." So for about six years I treated Mr. C. with medications, and in general he did acceptably well. He learned to walk more slowly; he resigned from some of the responsibilities that were stressing him, but he continued to have angina with emotional stress. Indeed, at his daughter's wedding, when he was overjoyed with her and his future son-in-law, he developed severe anginal pain, had to take three nitroglycerine tablets to ease it, and had to remove himself from the wedding procession because of recurrent chest pain. One early afternoon I got a phone call from Mrs. C. Mr. C. was having persistent chest pain, and no matter what he did and after four nitroglycerine tablets under the tongue, the pain persisted and was severe. On admission to the hospital it was clear that Mr. C. was having an episode of unstable angina (impending myocardial infarction). After stabilizing his condition medically he agreed to have emergency coronary angiography. The angiography revealed severe triple vessel atherosclerotic disease. He had agreed to the coronary angiography and now, after I explained his problem to him in detail, he agreed to having heart surgery with the aim of preventing any further heart muscle damage. The surgeon was able to effectively bypass the narrowings in the coronary arteries, Mr. C. made an uneventful recovery and, much to the delight of us all, his angina disappeared. When his second daughter married, he was able to engage fully in the proceedings without distress.

Dr. John Hunter, the famous English physician who is considered the father of surgery, suffered from angina pectoris. At that time the cause of angina was unknown and there was no treatment available. But Hunter knew the seriousness of his chest pain. He was quoted to have said, "My life is at the mercy of any rogue who chooses to provoke me." Sadly, Hunter died suddenly after a contentious medical meeting. His autopsy revealed severe coronary artery disease.

CHAPTER V.

CHEST PAINS|
—— NOT ORIGINATING FROM THE
HEARTor LUNGS|

A multitude of pains arise from the muscles, bones and nerves of the chest wall. Pains in the chest can originate from problems in the spine of the neck, and pains can present in the chest from problems under the diaphragm in the abdomen. Some of these pains are severe and merit attention because they hurt so much. Other pains warn of serious trouble, and therefore merit immediate medical attention. Many of these pains cause varying degrees of discomfort and call for non-urgent medical attention, but are not life threatening. In this chapter we will look at some classic examples of each.

Pains from the chest wall

The chest wall contains bones, cartilage, muscles, blood vessels and numerous nerves. The intercostal nerves originate in the spinal cord and an intercostal nerve passes under each rib (**Figure 9**). There are specific nerves supplying each of the chest wall muscles, and numerous pain fibers serve the skin itself.

Intercostal neuralgia

Intercostal neuralgia is pain that stems from the nerve between two ribs ("intercostal" means between ribs). It is invariably due to some kind of nerve inflammation, often due to a virus. The pain is sharp, may be quite severe, tends to be aggravated by breathing and may come and go. Sometimes it is severe, persistent and burning, as in herpes zoster, which is the technical name for "shingles." In this condition the pain tends to be persistent, the skin is often exquisitely sensitive to the slightest touch, and the pain invariably precedes the breaking out of a skin rash along the course of the nerve. Often the correct diagnosis awaits the breaking out of the rash. The rash and the intercostal neuralgia are due to a virus that affects the nerve, the same virus that causes chickenpox in children.

Dr. R.P., a 76-year old retired physician, was awakened in the middle of the night with a pain on the left side of his chest that gradually built in severity. On the next day the pain was intense. It swept around from the back to below the right

41

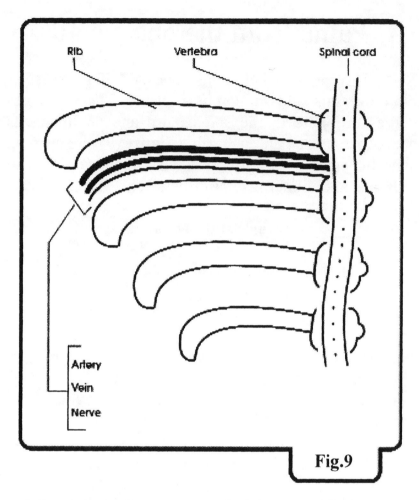

A diagram showing the nerve, artery, and vein between two ribs.

nipple area, had a rather burning quality, and was associated with increasing tenderness of the skin. His shirt against the side of his chest made him uncomfortable. Being a physician he knew that the pain was not from the heart, but because the pain was severe and worrisome he saw one of my partners that afternoon. We were not sure about the

42

origin of the pain, but the patient and my partner thought that it presented as a rather typical intercostal neuralgia. We all agreed that a rash might break out in the area of the pain. The prescribed pain medication helped somewhat and Dr. P. was started on an antiviral medication. Sure enough, a few days later he phoned to tell us that he had developed a rash along the path of the pain, a typical herpes zoster ("shingles").

Myositis involving the chest wall

There is a kind of chest wall pain that may be so severe it is called "Devil's grip." This severe pain usually occurs in epidemics and is due to a virus. It is also called Bornholm disease because it was first described on the island of Bornholm. It is thought to be due to a muscle inflammation, a "myositis," of the chest wall. The pain lasts for some days, with every breath hurting, and then it relents. In the unlucky few, it may return for another bout. The diagnosis is difficult unless the syndrome is seen in a number of people. This disease is easy to confuse with intercostal neuralgia, pleurisy or even a pain originating from the heart. The illness is self-limited, and I know of no particular treatment except pain relief.

Precordial catch

In my younger and thinner days I would sometimes get a severe sharp pain just below the left breast. At times bending over seemed to bring it on. It would come on suddenly, and every inspiration made it worse, so my immediate reaction was to breathe in a very shallow manner. On occasion forcing a deep breath in spite of the pain made it go away; otherwise it would last for some minutes. It tended to recur over the course of a few days, and then would not occur again for months. After a bout of the pain there sometimes remained a vague soreness in the left chest for one to two hours.

I was sure that this was not a serious pain, but when a few young patients, including my eldest daughter, described a strikingly similar pattern to me I became particularly interested and ended up collecting a series of cases that resulted in two medical publications. I named the syndrome the "precordial catch" because it felt like something got caught. The word "precordial" refers to the region over the heart and the lower part of the chest. Since my early papers, publications from other institutions have confirmed the occurrence and description of this syndrome. It is a completely benign event and though it may be quite discomfiting we still do not know what causes it.

Miss R.L., an 18-year old college student, saw me because of a recurrent terrible pain just under her left breast. It had started about nine days previously, the first episode occurring when she

44

was getting out of her friend's car. The pain was described as sudden in onset, severe, like a knife stabbing. When it hit she had to hold her breath because breathing in made the pain worse. Then she would breathe in a shallow manner for a few minutes until the pain went away. She had the idea that bending over sometimes brought on the pain. Sometimes standing very straight seemed to ease the pain. It kept occurring at odd times and had her quite worried about her heart. In addition to the sharp pains, she felt a vague aching in the left chest area. At no time had the pain occurred during the night or when she was lying down. Physical examination, an electrocardiogram and chest x-rays were normal. She was assured that she was experiencing a classic syndrome of precordial catch, that it was not serious, and that it would soon go away. One week later she phoned to tell me that the pain was "all gone." I explained to her that it might recur from time to time, and suggested she not worry about it.

Broken rib

A rib fracture can cause a mean pain. It usually follows a trauma, though may occur with such apparently benign episodes as severe coughing or heavy lifting. Splinting the area of the fracture often eases the pain, and makes breathing more comfortable. Usually rib fractures require no particular treatment, though on rare occasion a compound rib fracture can penetrate into the chest cavity and cause the collapse of a lung. Lung collapse is a serious complication, usually follows more severe injuries as might occur in an automobile accident, and demands emergency attention. Sometimes quite severe pain will follow a rib injury, even without a visible fracture. When rib pain persists, x-rays or other imaging techniques are indicated to rule out any underlying disease that is the cause of the pain. When rib pain and tenderness occur in the absence of a history of trauma a disease process involving the rib must be considered.

Xiphodynia

At the bottom of the breastbone there is a small bone that hangs down called the xiphoid process. It is of little importance, except that it sometimes becomes tender and patients like to press on it. Some people conclude that it is a tumor and head for the doctor. When it becomes sore, particularly if one keeps pressing on it, it can become a source of pain. The treatment is usually pretty straightforward - stop touching and pressing it and the pain will invariably disappear.

Chest pains from the spine

Pains from the spine of the neck

Problems such as arthritis or a ruptured disk between two vertebrae in the spine of the lower neck and the upper part of the back can cause chest pains. There is a cartilaginous pad, a so-called "disk," between each of the vertebra in the spine. A ruptured intervertebral disk occurs mainly in the neck and lower back area. Such a rupture produces an abnormal protrusion of the cartilage pad between two vertebrae (**Figure 10**) that presses on one or more nerve roots as they leave the spinal cord in such a way as to cause pain of varying degree and frequency.

Two important concepts mentioned before merit re-emphasis. The nerves passing around the chest wall all arise from the upper spinal cord (which is protected by the vertebral column of the neck and upper back). Pain is experienced at the point supplied by the nerve (where the nerve ends) in the tissue or organ, and not at the origin of the nerve. Thus, pain caused by severe arthritis in the neck can be experienced as pain across the shoulder and in the front of the upper chest. A typical example of such pain occurs in the person rear-ended in an automobile accident, who, suffering a whiplash injury, experiences severe muscle spasm in the neck and pain across the shoulder and in the upper front of the chest. Pain due to pathology of the upper spine, usually arthritis or a ruptured intervertebral disk, sometimes aggravated by osteoporosis in older persons, is usually recurrent. Such pain is precipitated by physical activity of certain kinds, peculiar positions, change in the weather and anything that causes muscle spasm including emotional stress.

Mr. A.R. weighed 240 lbs. A huge man, now 48

years old, he had played football as a tackle in high school and college. He played at a time in the history of the sport when using one's head-neck-body as a battering ram was still in vogue. He was knocked unconscious twice, and starting in his junior year in college he suffered neck pains that radiated across his left shoulder. He was treated with muscle relaxants and traction, and before each game he got a pain medication. Aspirin gave him some relief, as did heat and massage to relieve the muscle spasm.

When I saw Mr. R. he came in because of pain in the left upper chest and left shoulder, at times with considerable aching in the left elbow and forearm. The pain had become more severe in the preceding couple of months, and the patient was worried that some or all of the pain was coming from the heart because of the radiation of the pain to the left arm. Mr. R. was an avid cyclist, and at times the pain was quite bad when he was on his racing bike, but mainly it occurred when he was playing golf or gardening. An activity like raking leaves invariably brought on the pain. However, he could jog on his treadmill and have absolutely no pain, and fast walking on a level caused him no discomfort. His heart examination was normal, as was his blood pressure. All the arterial pulses were fine. An electrocardiogram and chest x-rays were normal, as were all his blood tests. A treadmill exercise test showed no abnormalities and revealed Mr. R. to be in excellent physical condition. He had no chest or arm pain during the test. We concluded that his problem was not cardiac, and that it was most likely from pathology in the neck. The striking aspect of the history was that only certain kinds of activity brought on the pain, whereas running did not do so. We referred him to a neurologist, whose studies revealed two large protruding cervical (neck) spine disks. He was treated with muscle relaxants and pain medication, but the pain became more severe. Eventually he had surgery on the ruptured intervertebral disks, and had marked relief from his shoulder and arm pain.

Interesting was a woman I saw who also had chest pain and pain across her left shoulder only with certain kinds of activities.

Mrs. T.U., a saleslady and homemaker, 44 years of age, was very worried about the pain she was getting high on the left side of her chest. Her mother died of a heart attack after having had angina pectoris for many years, and Mrs. U. was concerned that she had angina. She reported that the pain came on with physical activity. But on careful questioning it turned out that the pain occurred with particular activities, like sweeping the floor, reaching high to get things off shelves, making a bed, vacuuming the floor or bowling. But

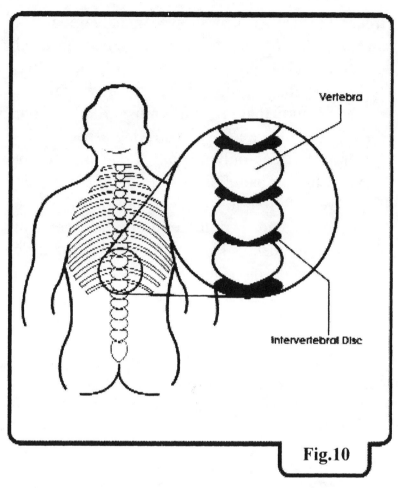

Vertebra

Intervertebral Disc

Fig.10

An intervertebral disc is present between each of the vertebra of the spine.

strenuous exercise such as fast walking, or walking uphill on her treadmill did not precipitate the pain. X-rays revealed severe arthritis of the vertebrae in the neck with narrowing of the intervertebral spaces. Studies proved her heart to be perfectly normal. An orthopedist prescribed muscle relaxants and anti-inflammatory agents and she had physical therapy with considerable improvement.

Pain in the shoulder

Pain in one of the shoulders is common. Usually the problem is a local one, like inflammation of a tendon, or arthritis, or tear of a rotator cuff. The pain in such situations is invariably related to movement of the shoulder. In older patients shoulder pain is a particular problem because if they restrict the use of the shoulder they are prone to develop a "frozen shoulder" that results in lasting limitation of motion at the shoulder joint.

Pain in the left shoulder area can be referred pain from the heart. Thus, angina pectoris, due to a decreased blood supply to the heart muscle with effort, can be manifest by pain in the left shoulder. As we will discuss later, the timing and circumstances of such pains are particularly important in making the diagnosis. To further complicate diagnosis, pain in the left shoulder can be due to inflammation or infection of the sac around the heart (the pericardial sac) or to pathology under the left side of the diaphragm.

When pain from the heart is referred to the left shoulder it is often associated with some discomfort in the left arm. We will discuss this topic at some length later, but an example here is worthwhile to emphasize its importance.

Mr. R.Z., a 48-year old lawyer who believed that exercise was a waste of time, was successful and very busy. He had many appointments and his life was becoming increasingly complicated with success. During the month previous to the time I saw him he had experienced left shoulder pain, really more of an aching discomfort, along with aching in the left elbow region, when he was rushed or angry. He had no such discomfort at any othertime, and though he was certain that the problem was an emotional one he decided that he better see me to check it out. The physical examination revealed his blood pressure to be moderately elevated to 160/100 mm Hg. The heart exam was unremarkable. All the usual tests were normal, including a resting electrocardiogram. After six minutes into a treadmill exercise test he developed a markedly abnormal electrocardiogram. He was admitted to the hospital, where a stress imaging study revealed a significant decrease in blood supply to a portion of the left ventricle with exercise. Coronary angiography revealed a marked narrowing (95 percent) of the proximal portion of the left anterior descending coronary artery. He was treated with angioplasty and the placement of a stent, and left the hospital in 2 days. He subsequently had no further shoulder or arm pain, and wisely decreased his loaded work schedule.

Pain in the left shoulder is a tricky symptom because it can mean so many things. In a later chapter we will provide additional examples of left shoulder pain of varying causes.

Pains from the esophagus

Pain from the lower esophagus

Pain from the lower esophagus, usually due to irritation or spasm, is sometimes initiated by regurgitation of stomach contents. It can be experienced as a burning sensation in the pit of the stomach (**Fig. 11**) that travels up under the breastbone ("heartburn") or as a tightness or constriction felt behind the lower part of the breastbone. At times it feels like pain that one experiences after swallowing a big chunk of cold ice cream. It is important to remember that the lower esophagus and the heart receive pain fibers from the same level of the spinal cord (**Figure 5**), and so it should not be surprising that the pain originating from the lower esophagus may be very difficult to differentiate from pain from the heart. Indeed, pain from the lower esophagus can be precipitated by such exercises as running, and that makes the differential diagnosis from heart pain particularly difficult.

The history provides important clues to pathology, the clues being mainly related to the company that the pain keeps. The patients with esophageal pain usually have a history of problems with certain foods. The pain often is precipitated by such foods as coffee, alcohol, or spicy dishes. A hot salsa or a bowl of hot chili is guaranteed to bring on the pain in susceptible individuals. The pain frequently relates to eating indiscretions, and is eased or relieved by antacids, milk, or such maneuvers as sipping hot water. I find the sipping hot water test particularly helpful, and usually hot water is readily available. Lower esophageal pains will be relieved by nitroglycerin administered under the tongue, just as is the pain of angina pectoris from the heart, because nitroglycerin relaxes the smooth muscle of the muscular lower esophagus. Patients with lower esophageal pains often have a hiatal hernia, which is a defect in the opening of the diaphragm, which allows part of an organ, usually the stomach, to slide up into the chest cavity. When an organ wanders in this way, lower esophageal spasm is more likely to occur. So-called "water brash" occurs with hiatal hernias and refers to sour disagreeable stomach contents that may regurgitate all the way to the mouth. This is more likely to happen when one is lying down. The tasting of water brash is a very uncomfortable experience that one is not likely to forget.

Obviously a lower esophageal pain syndrome does not protect a person from also having heart trouble; indeed, it is not rare for a person to have both conditions. A pressing, squeezing or constricting pain, sometimes a heaviness, in the lower middle of the front of the chest, with or without radiation, should lead a person to seek medical evaluation. Whether such pain reflects lower esophagus pathology or cardiac pathology, both are important and should be properly investigated.

Mr. T.T., a 38-year old vigorous carpenter, had played semi-professional baseball in his youth and remained physically very active. He still played basketball with a group of younger friends and worked out regularly at the local health club. Nevertheless, he continued to smoke cigarettes and maintained a substantial alcohol intake that included both beer and hard liquor. On occasion of his entering into a new business deal, a group of his friends took him out to dinner. His shrimp cocktail was followed with a big steak dinner and considerable beer and wine. That night, at about 3:00 AM, he was suddenly awakened with a terrible sour taste in the mouth due to regurgitation of some food, and he had a miserable burning pain in the pit of his stomach and behind the lower part of the breastbone. Sitting up and sipping some water made him a bit more comfortable. He awakened his wife, who thought he was having a heart attack and called 911. The paramedics took him to our hospital emergency room, where he was found to be tender in the upper mid abdomen. An electrocardiogram and various blood tests were normal. Specifically, tests for evidence of heart muscle injury were normal. He was kept in the hospital overnight and it was concluded that he had suffered no heart damage. A few days later upper endoscopy (looking down into the esophagus and stomach with a special tube device) by the gastroenterologist revealed a markedly inflamed lower esophagus and stomach. Mr. T. was advised to stop cigarettes, coffee and alcohol, and felt much better during the subsequent few weeks that he followed this advice.

Chest pains arising from pathology below the diaphragm

Irritation under the left side of the diaphragm

Over-eating can lead to a distended feeling in the abdomen that gives a vague chest discomfort and makes one vow to never eat like that again! Air pressing upward under the diaphragm may cause pain on the top of the shoulder.

Mrs. A.G., an executive secretary 48 years of age with high blood pressure, had recurrent left-sided abdominal pain. The diagnosis was unclear, and her gynecologist recommended laparoscopy, a technique of looking into the abdomen or pelvic area through a tiny incision with a "periscope-like" device, to examine the left ovary. The afternoon after the uneventful procedure, Mrs. G. phoned me complaining of severe pain on top of the left shoulder. I explained to her that the laparoscopic procedure required the injection of air into the abdominal cavity, and that she undoubtedly had some air pressing up under the left diaphragm. I assured her that this pain was not serious, that it would soon leave when the gas was absorbed, and that if she would lie down the air would shift and she would feel better. The next day the pain was gone and she felt fine.

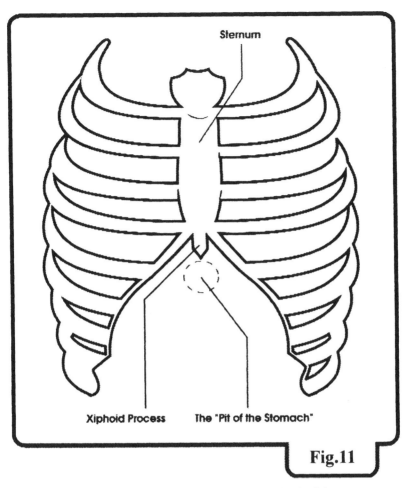

The area we know as "the pit of the stomach"(technically, "the epigastrium) is just below the xiphoid process.

Such a pain occurs after the injection of air into the abdominal cavity to facilitate a safe surgical procedure, and disappears when the gas is absorbed. Air can present under the diaphragm in more serious situations, such as the rupture of a hollow abdominal organ (for example, the stomach or colon) due to some pathology. Invariably such a rupture is an indication for emergency surgery.

A blood clot formed in the heart that gets loose and travels to impact the surface of the spleen - the spleen being tucked under the left diaphragm - may cause severe pain. The pain, located in the area of the lower left chest, is aggravated by inspiration (breathing in). The pain also can be felt on top of the left shoulder if the splenic injury causes irritation of the adjacent diaphragm. If the stomach slides up through a hiatal hernia and gets caught in the opening (a rare occurrence), severe lower chest pain may ensue. Though it is now fortunately a rare disease, an abscess under the diaphragm can cause pain on the side of the chest and in the shoulder, depending on where it is located.

Gall bladder colic

It used to be said that acute attacks of gall bladder colic, invariably related to the passage of a stone from the gall bladder into one of its ducts, could absolutely simulate pain from the heart. I have never personally seen this, but have seen instances in which pain between the shoulder blades was due to acute inflammation of the gall bladder (cholecystitis). Pancreatitis, an inflammation of the pancreas, can also give pain in this location. Both gall bladder and pancreatic disease cause epigastric pain, pain "in the pit of the stomach." (**Figure 11**).

CHAPTER VI

CHEST PAINS |
FROM THE
TRACHEA, BRONCHI & LUNGS |

Air is taken into the lungs (inhaled) by the expansion and lifting of the chest wall and the moving down of the muscular diaphragm. Air is pushed out of the lungs (exhaled) by the diaphragm moving up and the chest wall relaxing. Remember the old adage, "good air in, bad air out." The "good air" contains more oxygen, which is transferred to the blood in the small vessels (capillaries) from the tiny air sacs (alveoli) of the lung. The "bad air" contains more carbon dioxide, which is transferred from the capillaries to the alveoli to be breathed out into the atmosphere (see **Figure 12**).

The air comes into our bodies through the nose and mouth. Mouth breathing is more likely to occur during exertion, if the nose is congested and in persons that snore. From the nose or mouth the air passes through the pharynx into the trachea, the big round tube that you

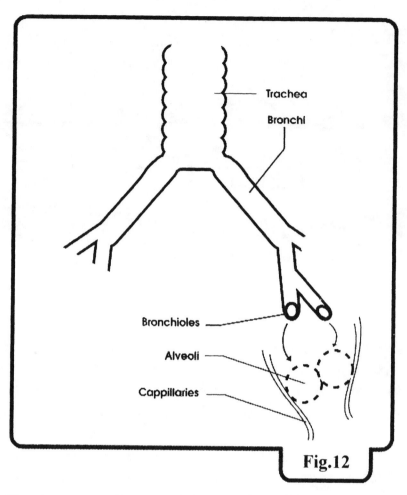

Fig.12

The trachea divides into the main bronchi, which eventually branch into the small bronchioles. These muscular small air passages pass the inhaled air to the delicate, thin-walled alveoli. The alveoli pass oxygenated blood to the thin-walled blood capillaries, and pick up carbon dioxide to be expelled.

can feel in the front of your neck. The trachea divides into the right and left bronchi, which in turn divide into smaller channels, then into bronchioles and finally to the little air sacs, the alveoli, where the gas exchanges actually take place. In essence the lungs consist of a myriad of tiny delicate air sacs that have conduits to deliver air to them. The function of the lungs in exchanging carbon dioxide for oxygen is critical to our survival; man cannot survive more than a few minutes without oxygen.

Chest pains arising from the trachea and bronchi

Tracheitis

Inflammation of the tracheal inner lining (**Figure 12**) is usually infectious in origin, but may be toxic as from inhaling smoke fumes. Indeed, some kinds of smoke fumes are very toxic, a hazard to which firefighters are exposed. Tracheal pain often is a sensation of rawness, and is most often located in the upper middle of the chest. The chest itself may feel heavy and congested. Tracheitis is usually part of an upper respiratory infection, as with a common cold or sore throat, and often presents in association with an acute bronchitis. A severe tracheobronchitis, involving the trachea and the bronchial tubes (for example, with the inhalation of toxic fumes), can cause shortness of breath.

Bronchitis

Most of us have had an acute bronchitis at one time or another. It is more common in places of poor air quality, with Mexico City being a classic example. I once developed a severe episode of bronchitis in rural New Guinea, where there was much smoke from open fires used for cooking. Bronchitis often follows a bout of the common cold, which progresses to a syndrome of cough, chest aching or heaviness, sometimes fever and sometimes chills. It is a frequent complication of influenza. Chronic bronchitis with acute flare-ups is common in cigarette smokers. Often there is a feeling of rawness in the upper mid chest as with tracheitis or tracheobronchitis. The cough may be so severe as to cause chest soreness, usually on both sides, and in the lower chest. The "pain" of bronchitis is mainly a combination of the rawness and chest soreness related to coughing. As noted before, inflammation of bronchi is often associated with inflammation of the trachea that leads to them. Bronchitis may precede pneumonia.

Chest pains from the lung

Pleurisy

It is of interest that though the lungs are critical to our survival, they contain few pain fibers. Pain can arise from the trachea and bronchi and from the inner lining of the chest wall. The surface of the lung, the visceral pleura, has relatively few pain fibers, but the

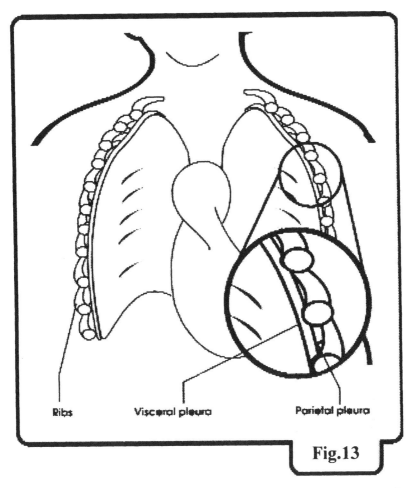

Ribs   Visceral pleura   Parietal pleura

Fig.13

The pleura is the thin smooth layer that covers the inside of the chest wall (parietal pleura) and the surface of the lung (visceral pleura).

parietal pleura, the inner lining of the chest cavity against which the lung expands, is abundantly supplied with pain fibers **(Figure 13)**. Pleurisy, an inflammation of the surface lining of the lung and the adjacent lung tissue, can be associated with considerable pain. The pain is due to involvement of the parietal pleura, is almost always on the side of the chest, is sharp, often severe, and invariably is made worse by breathing in (inspiration) when the surface of the lung slides along the inside of the chest wall (**Figure 13**). Patients with pleurisy tend to limit breathing to short, shallow respirations to ease the pain and the rate of breathing is usually increased. Pleurisy, which is most often infectious in origin due to a virus or bacteria, usually is associated with some degree of underlying pneumonia (inflammation of the lung itself). We don't see as much pleurisy now as in the past, which may be due to the rather extensive use of antibiotics or to other unidentified causes.

John T.O., a 16-year old high school student, visited the school nurse with the complaint "of feeling rotten." He had a slight fever, complained of some chills, and said he had a bad pain on the right side of his chest. He reported, "Every time I take a deep breath the pain is terrible." Because John looked quite sick, his mother was called and she took him to their family physician. The doctor made a diagnosis of acute pleurisy after hearing a crackling sound, a friction rub, over the right lower chest. A "friction rub" is a sound like that made by rubbing two pieces of leather together. A chest x-ray showed a small amount of fluid in the right lower chest, consistent with pleurisy. In a few days the pain disappeared.

Pleurisy is usually a benign condition, but at times it results from serious pathology. A cancer may involve

64

the pleura and cause pain. Pleurisy is often associated with pneumonia. It sometimes occurs after heart operations. Pleuritic pain can be important in pointing to serious, even life-threatening, conditions such as pulmonary embolization (see below).

Pneumonia

Pneumonia, an inflammation within the lung, often follows an upper respiratory infection, usually is infectious in origin (caused by a virus or bacteria), and may involve various parts of the lung. Central pneumonia, in which there is no involvement of the surface of the lung, may be completely painless or may be associated with vague chest heaviness. Pneumonia that involves the surface of the lung is associated with the pain of pleurisy, which is sharp, may be quite severe, and is made worse by breathing in. The clinical picture usually includes fever, chills, and cough, but exceptions are many depending on the resistance of the patient, the virulence of the infecting organism, and the location of the infection. Patients with pneumonia usually have an increased breathing rate and breathe in a shallow pattern.

Pulmonary embolism

Mr. J.S., a 42-year old machinery salesman, came to the office very anxious and complaining of left chest pain. He felt weak and "out of sorts."

He was worried about his heart. The pain had started the preceding day, came on suddenly, and made him breathe as shallowly as possible because every deeper breath caused excruciating pain. On the previous night, after the pain had started, he coughed up some pinkish looking sputum. Five days previously he had returned from a business trip to Japan. On physical examination he had some tenderness in the calf of the right leg. His heart rate was moderately rapid at 100 beats per minute. His breathing was shallow. The breath sounds were decreased at the left lung base and some dry rales (crackling sounds) were heard. We hospitalized Mr. S. with the diagnosis of an acute pulmonary embolism. The diagnosis was confirmed with chest x-rays and a special kind of imaging study (CT scan). An ultrasound study of the legs revealed a blood clot in a vein of the right calf.

A pulmonary embolus is a blood clot that obstructs a branch of the pulmonary artery. The pulmonary artery is the large vessel that carries blood from the right ventricle to the lung (**Figure 4**). The pulmonary embolus that this patient suffered is a serious condition and merits prompt attention. A large clot suddenly occluding an artery to the lung can cause sudden death. Making the diagnosis is important for two main reasons: first, to treat the embolization and dissolve the blood clot and second, to prevent further clots traveling to the lung. Such clots can form in the antechamber of the right ventricle (the right atrium) or in veins that send blood to the right ventricle. A blood clot in a leg vein or, in women a blood clot in the pelvic area, can only pass to the right ventricle and then to the lung. Such clots are more likely to occur in persons with varicose veins of the legs and after long periods of sitting, as with a long plane ride. There is some reason to believe that sitting with the legs crossed makes a clot formation more likely.

Patients suffering a pulmonary embolus often feel anxious. The anxiety may have a physiological origin and may be a clue to the diagnosis. The kind of pain that occurs with pulmonary embolization depends upon what part of the lung is involved. When the outer part of the lung is affected, the chest pain is usually sudden in onset, is sharp and severe, is likely to be associated with cough and is made worse by breathing in. The pain is similar to that of pleurisy. Large clots can be associated with sweating, pallor, rapid shallow breathing, an irregular pulse, shortness of breath, a fall in blood pressure and even shock. Coughing up blood sometimes occurs. Fever may occur and the clinical picture may simulate pneumonia. Clots that affect lung tissue not on the surface may cause only chest aching, pressure or heaviness that is not much affected by breathing. They are often associated with rapid breathing. Pulmonary emboli frequently precipitate some heart irregularities.

Congestive heart failure

The classic definition of heart failure defines it as the inability of the heart to pump sufficient blood to meet the needs of the body. We now know that heart failure is associated with important hormonal and chemical changes. Such changes include kidney function effects that lead to salt and water retention and to excessive sympathetic nervous system stimulation of the heart.

Heart failure with congestion of the lungs can cause a sensation of heaviness in the front of the chest that is sometimes difficult to differentiate from a heart muscle injury. Congestive heart failure will sometimes cause the patient to complain of a "choking sensation." This was the term originally used by Heberden when he first described angina pectoris.

Heart failure is usually associated with other symptoms and signs that help differentiate it from angina, though it should be noted that anginal pain can occur in the presence of heart failure. Decreased blood supply to the heart muscle due to atherosclerotic disease of the coronary arteries is a major cause of heart failure, as is chronic high blood pressure. A previous or present myocardial infarction (heart attack) with loss of heart muscle predisposes to heart failure that may come on suddenly or gradually. Heart failure may also be caused by infection of the heart muscle and by various diseases that interfere with its function, such as diseases that injure the heart valves. Rheumatic fever, the major cause of heart valve injury, is less and less common in the Western world, undoubtedly due to improved socioeconomic conditions and antibiotic treatment of streptococcus sore throats and scarlet fever, conditions that precede it.

Heart failure is usually associated with shortness of breath with physical activity, increased shortness of breath and discomfort when lying flat (due to lung congestion), rapid respirations, palpitations, swelling of the ankles, abdominal discomfort, and distinctive findings on physical examination.

Mr. T.Z., a 74-year old retired tailor, came to the office complaining of a sensation of heaviness in the front of the chest present for 4 days and increasing shortness of breath. He couldn't lie down because he then became very short of breath, so he had been sleeping in an easy chair. He noticed his heart pounding. He felt weak, even going to the bathroom was an effort, and he felt like he was going to die. Five years previously he had suffered a heart attack and subsequent angina. About one year after the heart attack he had coronary angiography that visualized narrowings in two of his coronary arteries. He then had balloon dilation of these narrowings (angioplasty). He felt quite well after that for about five years, was able to be reasonably active and only had angina when he was rushing, as when he was late to get to an appointment. We hospitalized him when he again developed heart failure with increasing fatigue and shortness of breath. Cardiac catheterization showed that he had severe atherosclerosis ("hardening of the arteries") of all three major coronary artery branches. A portion of the left ventricle was not contracting at all (the old heart attack area) and another substantial area was contracting rather weakly but did improve when certain drugs were administered. An imaging study confirmed the poor contraction of the left ventricle of the heart. He was vigorously treated with diuretics and medications to decrease the work of the heart and improved substantially.

Mr. Z. agreed to have the coronary bypass surgery that was recommended. The surgeon was able to bypass all three major coronary artery branches. The patient did well and went home on the 6th day after surgery. Though he still required medication for his heart disease after surgery, he no longer had the choking sensation in the chest with exertion and was able to function comfortably. A repeat study of his heart muscle function revealed the left ventricular contraction significantly improved over the findings before the heart operation.

A different cause for heart failure is seen with rheumatic heart disease, which is statistically more frequent in women.

Mrs. M.L. was first seen in our offices when she was 42 years old. She gave a history of having had rheumatic fever when she was age 12 years, at which time she was kept in bed for one month. She felt well after that and was able to keep up with all the other kids, but she was left with a heart murmur. Her major complaint was shortness of breath on relatively mild exertion and chronic fatigue, both symptoms having progressed in the preceding year. When I examined her she had the classic murmur of narrowing (stenosis) of the valve (mitral valve) between the left atrium (the antechamber to the left ventricle), and the left ventricle. An echocardiogram confirmed the presence of a moderately severe stenosis of the mitral valve.

The mitral valve separates the left antechamber of the heart from the main left pumping chamber, the left ventricle, that pumps blood to the body (**see figure 5**). Mitral stenosis causes the blood to back up into the lung and the output of blood to the body is impaired.

Mrs. L. did well with medical management until 13 years after first she was seen. At the age of 55 years, she had developed an irregular heart rhythm and complained of increasing fatigue and shortness of breath. When she exerted herself, like making a bed or vacuuming or working in the garden she developed a heaviness on the chest with severe shortness of breath that made it necessary for her to stop and rest. Various studies, including an electrocardiogram and an echocardiogram, confirmed that Mrs. L. had progressed to a severe narrowing at the mitral valve. Heart catheterization and coronary angiography revealed her coronary arteries to be normal. She had a fracture (forced opening) of the mitral valve by passing a special type of balloon catheter to the site of the valve and improved quickly and markedly. Then, after about three more years she began to have trouble again and now it was decided to replace her mitral valve. She had the surgery with the placement of a mechanical valve to replace her diseased mitral valve, her recovery was uneventful, and since then she has been feeling quite well. Because of her relatively young age and because she had an irregular heart rhythm that required her being on anticoagulant therapy, a metallic prosthesis was used by the surgeon. She has had no further chest heaviness and shortness of breath with routine household chores.

CHAPTER VII

CHEST PAINS |
ARISING FROM THE
AORTA |

The aorta is the large blood vessel that arises from the left ventricle of the heart (**Figure 4**). The left ventricle pumps blood through the aorta to all the tissues of the body except the lungs. Arising from the aorta are important arteries that provide blood to the heart itself (the coronary arteries), the brain (the carotid and vertebral arteries), and all the other organs of the body including the muscles.

Dissection of the aorta

The aorta is subject to atherosclerosis ("hardening of the arteries") and to various imperfections that form on its inner surface. It is subject to the relatively high pressure with which the blood is pumped into it from the left ventricle. Most patients with this condition "dissection of the aorta" are those with untreated or inadequately treated high blood pressure. Dissection of

73

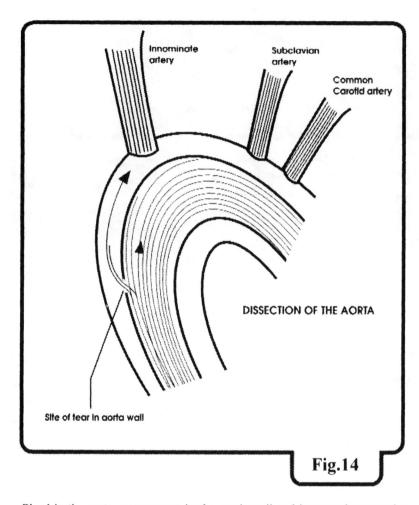

Innominate artery

Subclavian artery

Common Carotid artery

DISSECTION OF THE AORTA

Site of tear in aorta wall

Fig.14

Blood in the aorta enters a tear in the aortic wall and burrows between the aortic layers. The dissection may occlude various arteries arising from aorta.

the aorta, a serious pathology that is a threat to life, occurs when the blood within the aorta works its way into a defect in its wall and then burrows along between the layers of the wall of the aorta (**Figure 14**). As the blood burrows along it can obstruct various vessels that arise from the aorta. The dissection itself can cause considerable pain. The symptoms and signs that occur depend on which vessels are obstructed by the dissection. Blocking of a coronary artery will lead to a heart attack (myocardial infarction). Occlusion of a vessel to the brain can cause a stroke. Obstruction of an artery that supplies the intestine may lead to gangrene of a portion of it. The treatment depends on the circumstances, and will vary from an intensive medical approach to emergency surgery.

Patients having a dissection of the aorta usually experience excruciating, tearing pain. The pain may start between the shoulder blades or in front of the chest. At times it is so severe and sudden in onset that the patient literally falls to the knees or collapses. The pain can shift from one place to another as the dissection progresses. It may move upward, and then pass downward, depending on the area of dissection and which organs are involved. Dissection of the aorta is a grave emergency calling for immediate hospitalization and special diagnostic studies to define the area of dissection and its origin.

Mr. T.O., a retired railroad worker 68 years of age with a long history of high blood pressure, often would neglect to take his medicine. A recent blood pressure check at the blood pressure machine in the local grocery store of 180/105 mm Hg led him to make an appointment to come to the office the following week. He was standing on a street corner waiting for the light to change when he experienced a sudden excruciating pain between the shoulder blades that knocked him to his knees. The policeman at the corner called an ambulance and Mr. O. was taken to our hospital emergency room. On arrival his blood pressure was 190/110 mm Hg and he described terrible pain between the shoulder blades in the back that had also radiated to the front of the chest. A diagnosis of dissection of the aorta was confirmed with ultrasound studies. An electrocardiogram and blood enzymes gave evidence of an acute myocardial infarction. Mr. O. fortunately recovered from the acute dissection and the complicating heart attack after vigorous treatment to lower the blood pressure and maintain it well within the normal range.

Patients with Marfan's syndrome, a congenital condition associated with degeneration of the middle layer of the aorta, are particularly prone to aortic dissection. This may occur as a lethal catastrophe in young patients. Prophylactic surgical replacement of a portion of the aorta is sometimes a consideration in these young patients.

Aneurysm of the aorta

Areas of weakness in the aorta can bulge out, just as the inner tubes in the old tires used to do, and they can rupture. Aneurysms of the aorta (**Figure 15**) are usually due to weakness of the wall caused by atherosclerosis or syphilis, though fortunately we almost never see the latter anymore. Aneurysms occur in the aorta in the chest and in the abdomen. The rupture of an aortic

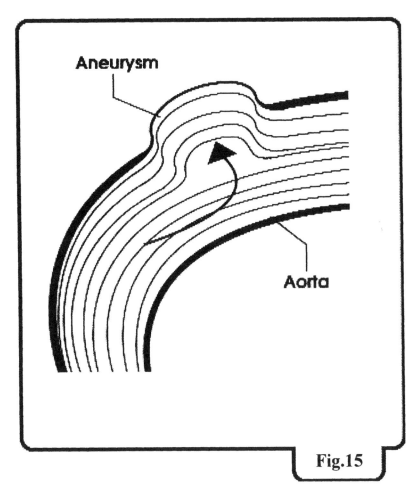

Aneurysm

Aorta

Fig.15

A aneurysm of the aorta is a bulging out at an area of aortic
wall weakness.

aneurysm in either location is a catastrophe and calls for
emergency surgery, but the results of such emergency
surgery are poor. I have a patient who survived such a
catastrophe with rupture of an abdominal aneurysm
thanks to prompt surgery, but another patient who had a
rupture of an aneurysm of the aorta in the chest ended up

77

with a bad stroke. Because of the poor results of emergency surgery after an aneurysm ruptures, when larger aneurysms are diagnosed prophylactic surgery is usually recommended. Smaller aneurysms are carefully monitored at regular intervals with ultrasound or special x-ray techniques (e.g. computerized tomography). Treatment options are both medical and surgical. Medical treatment is directed to reducing elevated blood pressures to low normal ranges and keeping the pressure on the wall of the aneurysm down. Surgical treatment generally replaces that section of the aorta with a special kind of tubular graft. This approach has a reasonable risk and the results are quite good. Recently, a new technique of treating abdominal aneurysms was developed. It consists of placing a special kind of retaining cylinder into the aorta from an artery in the groin, thus avoiding an abdominal incision.

The pain of an intact aortic aneurysm varies from no discomfort at all to a burning, persistent, debilitating pressure. The pain usually is related to what organs or nerves are being compressed by the bulging aneurysm.

Mr. C.A., age 68-years, was getting vague abdominal distress and nausea after eating, particularly after larger meals. A CT scan of the abdomen showed a gall bladder full of stones and an abdominal aortic aneurysm of moderate size. We thought his symptoms were related to the gall bladder. He had an uneventful removal of the gall bladder via a laparoscopic surgical approach, and thereafter his abdominal symptoms disappeared.

We followed a program of regular CT scans to watch the size of the abdominal aortic aneurysm. It slowly got larger, and by the time Mr. A. was 74 years of age it had gotten disturbingly large. The aneurysm was surgically cut out and that portion of the aorta was replaced with a graft. Mr. A. made a smooth recovery and has done well since.

CHAPTER VIII

CHEST PAINS |
FROM THE
HEART & PERICARDIUM |

Chest pains arising from the pericardium

Pericarditis

The pericardium is the translucent sac around the heart (**Figure 16**). It has abundant pain fibers and is a source of pain under certain circumstances. In the more recent past pericardial disease due to infection has decreased in frequency. The most frequent cause for pain arising from the pericardium is infection that involves the sac and the surface of the heart, with viral infections undoubtedly now being the most frequent cause. Years ago tuberculosis was the main cause of pericarditis, but it is now infrequently encountered. Sometimes the cause of pain arising from the pericardial sac is not infection, but rather an irritation to the

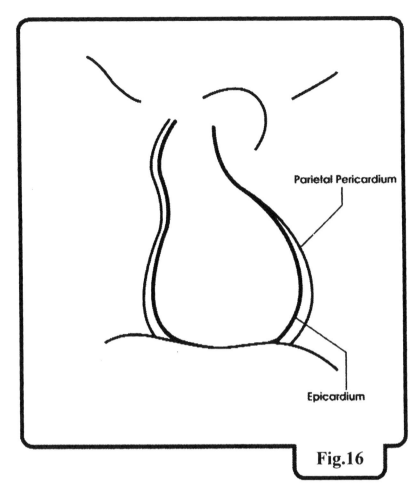

Parietal Pericardium

Epicardium

Fig.16

The parietal pericardium is the "sac" around the heart. There is normally a small amount of fluid in the pericardial space. Another term for the epicardium, the thin lining over the heart, is "visceral pericardium."

pericardium, as can occur with bleeding into the pericardial sac. More exotic causes are seen from time to time. Certain so-called "autoimmune diseases" are associated with pericarditis. These diseases, examples being lupus erythematosus and rheumatoid arthritis, are

81

thought to be due to the body inappropriately attacking some of its own cells and structures as if they were foreign invaders.

The pain of pericarditis is quite variable. If the inflammation involves the lower part of the pericardium that sits on the diaphragm the pain may be referred to the top of the left shoulder. Usually the pain that occurs is dull, aching and persistent. It may wax and wane in intensity, and at times is very uncomfortable. It most frequently is felt in the front of the chest or to the side, is made worse by lying down and may be eased by bending forward when in the sitting position. On occasion the pain is made worse by swallowing as the food or liquid passes the area where the heart leans on the esophagus.

Episodes of acute pericarditis are often associated with pleurisy (a pleuropericarditis), and then breathing in, particularly a deep inspiration, makes the pain worse. Patients with this condition often feel and look ill. Some degree of fever is common. On occasion the pericarditis is recurrent, coming back after an interval when the patient felt well.

Pericarditis may complicate an acute myocardial infarction ("heart attack") and is not rare after heart surgery. A rubbing sound (a friction rub) may be heard with the stethoscope in such circumstances. Pericarditis due to a virus or blood in the pericardial sac is usually a relatively benign condition, but at times is followed by a marked laying down of fibrous tissue ("scarring") in the pericardial sac. This pathology, called "adhesive" or "constrictive" pericarditis, may seriously interfere with heart function by interfering with blood flowing back into the heart from the large veins. When necessary, surgical removal of such scar tissue surrounding the heart is successfully accomplished.

Pericarditis has to be differentiated from a heart attack (acute myocardial infarction). Usually the differential diagnosis is straightforward, but at times it is difficult inasmuch as the pain of pericarditis may closely simulate that of a heart muscle injury. And, as noted, pericarditis may be a complication of a myocardial infarction.

Chest pains arising from the heart

Heart trouble worries many of us. We know that the heart is a major Achille's heel in our Society. We know that heart disease is serious and that the heart is an organ that can be associated with sudden death. In the modern era of medicine we should also be aware that there is a great deal that can be done to prevent and treat heart disease, so making the correct diagnosis has particularly large dividends. We can think of the heart as consisting of four major divisions:

1. The two muscular heart chambers(ventricles) that pump the blood to the lungs and the body and their two antechambers (atria).

2. The coronary arteries that supply blood to the heart muscle.

3. The impulse conduction system that controls the heart rhythm and rate (**Figure 17**).

4. The valves that direct the proper flow of the blood in the heart.

Disease of any of these four anatomical constituents, or a combination of them, can cause pain in the chest. The emphasis will be on those conditions that are important and common.

Diseases of the heart muscle

Hypertrophic cardiomyopathies
Such diseases of the heart muscle are not rare, and are sometimes associated with sudden death. Hypertrophic cardiomyopathy, a marked thickening due to disorganized muscle cell overgrowth, may cause vague chest discomfort. The discomfort is generally not sufficient to demand medical attention. On occasion it can lead to vague chest pain with exertion. Sometimes it is associated with feelings of heaviness or constriction in the front of the chest and at times palpitations are experienced.

John G.S. was a tall, lanky, African-American 22-year old, a superb basketball player who was already being scouted by National Basketball

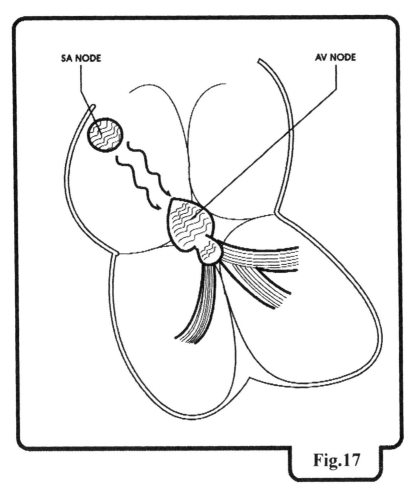

SA NODE

AV NODE

Fig.17

The "electrical system" of the heart. The impulse starts in the SA node, travels down to the AV node, passes down to an area called the Bundle of His, and then is spread via the bundle branches to the right and left ventricles.

Association teams. His family wanted him to finish college, but the contract offers he had received were quite exciting. He was playing his usual active, skilled game against a rival college when he suddenly collapsed on the basketball court. He was given immediate cardiopulmonary resuscitation (CPR) and rushed to the hospital, where he was pronounced dead. His family and friends were devastated. His mother and father assured us that he had never complained of any chest pain, though his girlfriend said that he sometimes talked about a vague chest heaviness that he dismissed as muscular aching.

An autopsy revealed marked thickening of the wall of the left ventricle and the septum (separating muscle and tissue between the two ventricles) consistent with hypertrophic cardiomyopathy. Study of the patient's two brothers and one sister showed echocardiographic evidence of suggestive hypertrophic cardiomyopathy in one of the brothers.

Hypertrophic cardiomyopathy is probably congenital in most instances, an inherited family trait, and can be treated if diagnosed early enough. A family history of this kind of problem calls for medical attention. Close relatives of a person with hypertrophic cardiomyopathy always should be checked. In the future, genetic profiling will likely prove helpful in this kind of disease.

Dilated cardiomyopathies

This condition is in some ways the opposite of the enlargement of the heart muscle seen in the hypertrophic state. Here the heart becomes "weak and flabby" and its ability to pump blood is seriously impaired. Sometimes a dilated cardiomyopathy is seen as a rather acute condition, for example, following heart muscle inflammation that occurs secondary to a viral infection. Such a heart muscle injury can lead to a dilated cardiomyopathy and even the need for a heart transplant. But usually dilated cardiomyopathy is gradual in onset, the classic cause being alcoholism. The main symptoms in this condition are related to failure of the heart to adequately pump blood to the body. They include shortness of breath, weakness, fluid retention and abnormal heart rhythms. Chest pain is generally not an important part of the picture, though complaints of a sensation of chest heaviness do occur. Whether this symptom comes from the heart or from the fluid accumulation in the lungs may be difficult to discern.

Mr. T.U., a 32-year old Mexican-American construction worker, had been married about three weeks when he complained to his wife of shortness of breath. The shortness of breath was associated with a feeling of heaviness in the chest and he felt "skipped beats" quite often. The shortness of breath got worse, and when I saw him some two weeks later he was short of breath on minimal exertion. Walking from the waiting room to my office made him so short of breath that he had trouble talking. On examination he was unable to lie flat because of breathing difficulty. The neck veins were distended, his ankles were swollen, he had evidence of fluid in the lungs and the liver was enlarged. The heart examination revealed a 3rd heart sound consistent with heart failure and he had many premature heart beats. An electrocardiogram was markedly abnormal and consistent with a myocarditis (inflammation of the heart muscle). Chest x-rays revealed the heart to be markedly enlarged. Mr. U. was hospitalized and treatment made him moderately more comfortable. Heart catherization and coronary angiography revealed normal coronary arteries and a markedly enlarged "flabby" heart with very poor heart function. Mr. U. was referred for cardiac transplantation, which was successfully accomplished about one month later. Study of the diseased heart revealed microscopic changes consistent with an acute viral infection. About four years after his heart transplantation he was doing well and engaged in a modified work schedule.

Myocarditis

Myocarditis is an inflammation of the heart muscle, caused by infection or some toxic substance. Viruses are the most common cause, but certain drugs can also cause significant heart muscle inflammation. Some of the drugs used to treat cancer may cause heart muscle damage and that is why oncologists will carefully monitor the heart status of patients getting such drugs. Myocarditis often occurs in acute rheumatic fever, which is now uncommon in the United States but is still common in India and in developing nations. A degree of heart muscle inflammation is always associated with pericarditis (inflammation of sac around the heart). Myocarditis may cause chest pain which generally is described as a feeling of heaviness in the front of the chest. If associated with a pericarditis, the pain may be the more compelling kind characteristic of pericarditis. Myocarditis can be a rather difficult diagnosis to make. At times a biopsy from the inside of the ventricular muscle is helpful. This procedure is done through a catheter passed into the heart from a blood vessel in the groin, and though it sounds formidable it is relatively quite safe. As noted with the patient presented previously, myocarditis can result in a dilated cardiomyopathy.

Diseases of the coronary arteries

The coronary arteries arise from the base of the aorta and provide oxygenated blood to the heart muscle. The heart is appropriately selfish in that it feeds itself before pumping blood to the rest of the body. There are two main coronary arteries, and the left one branches close to its origin into two large vessels (**Figure 18**). Doctors generally refer to the three major coronary artery branches. These coronary arteries are located on the surface of the heart, and supply the heart muscle through a myriad of smaller branches that penetrate down into it. It is the large coronary arteries on the heart surface that are peculiarly susceptible to atherosclerosis. Atherosclerosis ("hardening of the arteries") generally consists of one or more plaques on the inner surface of the blood vessel that project into its lumen (the channel of the blood vessel) (**Figure 19**). The typical plaque includes cholesterol, smooth muscle, various white blood cells, blood platelets, scar tissue and calcium. When an atherosclerotic plaque ruptures, or when its surface lining erodes and breaks open, a blood clot forms at the site of the rupture. Such a blood clot superimposed on the atherosclerotic plaque markedly or totally obstructs the flow of blood in the vessel. The result is a myocardial infarction (heart attack) or a lesser degree of heart muscle injury.

When atherosclerosis, either localized or involving more of the inside of the arteries, progresses to become severe enough, it interferes with blood flow just as excessive deposits on the inside of pipes slows water to your house. When an atherosclerotic plaque markedly narrows the channel of the coronary artery, then interference with blood flow may occur under certain circumstances. For example, anginal pain, due to decreased blood supply to a part of the heart muscle, may occur when the person walks up stairs or rushes to catch a bus. Large plaques with more calcium and scar tissue interfere with blood flow, however, the smaller, softer plaques with more cholesterol in their core are the ones more likely to rupture and lead to local clot formation and myocardial infarction.

Physicians talk about "invasive" and "non-invasive" treatments of atherosclerotic coronary artery disease. "Invasive" treatment consists of such procedures as balloon dilation of the narrowed area (angioplasty) and placing a stent to help keep the area open. This treatment is directed at improving the blood supply to an area of heart muscle. "Non-invasive" treatment directed at the atherosclerotic plaque involves the use of drugs to stabilize it and minimize the risk of rupture or progression. With the use of some of the newer drugs the hope is to pull cholesterol out of the plaque.

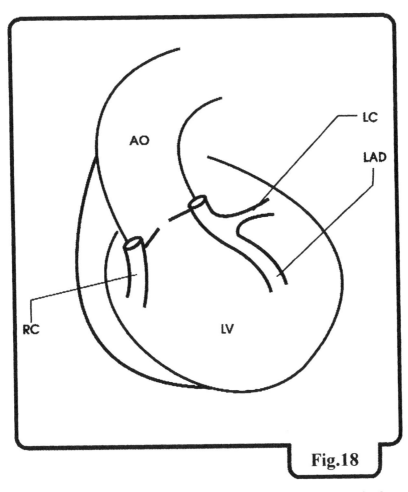

The blood circulation to the heart muscle. The coronary arteries arise from the base of the aorta (AO). LV - left ventricle. LAD - left anterior descending coronary artery. LC -left circumfles artery. RC - right coronary artery.

Myocardial infarction

When the blood supply via a coronary artery to an area of heart muscle is cut off, the result is injury to the muscle and the eventual death of the muscle so deprived

91

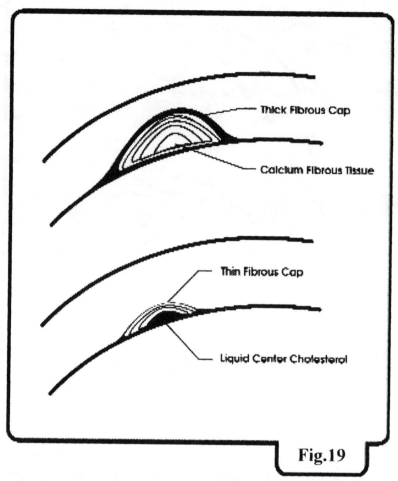

Labels in figure:
- Thick Fibrous Cap
- Calcium Fibrous Tissue
- Thin Fibrous Cap
- Liquid Center Cholesterol

Fig.19

Atherosclerotic plaques. The top figure shows a 'hard' plaque with a thick fibrous cap. This is a relatively stable plaque. The bottom figure shows a 'soft' plaque, with a thin fibrous cap and a large liquid center. The latter plaque is more susceptible to rupture or cap erosion.

of oxygen and nourishment. Doctors name this event an "acute myocardial infarction," the term that comes closest to the lay descriptive term of "heart attack." The body deals with the death of an area of heart muscle by replacing the dead muscle with scar tissue. Usually the resultant scar is stronger than the surrounding muscle, but it does not contribute to the work of the heart to propel blood.

The usual image of the "typical heart attack" victim is a middle-aged man who sports all the risk factors, including cigarette smoking, elevated blood pressure, high cholesterol, obesity, a sedentary lifestyle and a family history of diabetes. But the exceptions to this so-called "typical" scenario are very many. Indeed, heart attacks that are due to coronary artery atherosclerosis are seen in men in their thirties, and in women. Indeed, as we have noted before, women should pay attention to their typical and atypical pains, and physicians must understand that women of all ages get coronary artery disease. Women taking the birth control pill who are cigarette smokers are particularly vulnerable to heart attacks. Cocaine users are also at added risk.

It is worth re-stating that for many years doctors firmly believed that menstruating women were very unlikely to have significant atherosclerosis and its resultant arterial disease. Indeed, it was the general belief that pre-menopausal women never suffered myocardial infarction ("heart attack"). We now know that this entrenched belief was wrong; menstruating women do have atherosclerosis, and those with diabetes are particularly vulnerable.

Chest pain is usual with an acute "heart attack," and varies from mild to terribly severe. The pain is usually in the middle of the chest, behind the breastbone, and may radiate to the left shoulder and arm. Sometimes it radiates to the neck and jaw, it may radiate to the throat, and on occasion it is felt between the shoulder blades in the back. Sometimes the pain is felt only in the left shoulder and arm. On rare occasion it is in the "pit of the stomach" (the upper middle part of the abdomen) and can be confused with an abdominal condition. I can recall one patient who had pain to the right of the breastbone and in the right shoulder with his heart attack, though that is most unusual. It is not unusual to have a history of a milder chest pain preceding the more severe one, sometimes by as long as two weeks.

The chest pain is accompanied by various general bodily symptoms, particularly when the heart attack is more severe. The blood pressure may fall. Usually the heart rate increases, but with certain kinds of heart attacks the heart rate slows. Often the patient is pale, feels weak, and complains of lightheadedness. A cold sweat may occur, and is associated with a rather weak pulse. But even without any of these complicating symptoms, the patient is an emergency and he or she and relatives must act appropriately by seeking immediate medical attention. There is much to do to reduce complications and the risk of death from an acute myocardial infarction; it is foolhardy to delay getting proper help.

Mr. A.G., a 55-year old energetic manager of a department store, was chairing a morning sales meeting when he developed an increasingly uncomfortable pain in the middle of the chest. It reminded him of a similar milder pain he had felt a week before. At first he thought it was indigestion, but it kept getting worse and became associated with an aching in his left elbow and wrist. He felt rather weak, became lightheaded and told his assistant that he would have to end the meeting because he felt ill. She observed that he looked pale, helped him to an easy chair and gave him some water to drink. Mr. G. said that the pain was pretty bad and so without further discussion the floor manager called 911. The paramedics started Mr. G. on oxygen and took him to our hospital, where he was started on medications to decrease formation of blood clot in the coronary artery. In the cardiac catheterization laboratory, coronary angiography (visualization of the coronary arteries) revealed a severe narrowing in the mid portion of the left anterior descending coronary artery. The physician dilated the lesion with a balloon catheter and placed a stent. Studies revealed that the patient had sustained a moderate sized heart attack, but the opening of the affected artery by dilation and stenting undoubtedly prevented more heart damage or death.

As I have stressed, a myocardial infarction is due to the loss of blood supply to an area of the heart muscle. Untreated, the result is the death of the blood-deprived muscle and its replacement by a scar. Though the scar usually can handle the normal pressure build up caused by contraction of the ventricular muscle, it is of no help in pumping blood to the body. It is clear, therefore, that every effort should be made to prevent heart attacks and the loss of heart muscle. In patients experiencing a heart attack we make every effort to limit the extent of the heart muscle loss, but obviously it would be better to prevent any muscle loss in the first place.

Angina pectoris

Angina pectoris is the classic pain produced when some part of the heart muscle is not getting enough blood for the task or situation at hand. Consequently, the pain invariably occurs when an added load is placed on the heart muscle, such added loads being physical or emotional. It is apparent that anyone experiencing chest pain with physical or emotional stress should seek medical counsel.

Mrs. T.F., an active librarian 64 years of age, was very regular in her habits and always caught the 8:15 A.M. bus to work. The bus stop was 2 blocks from her house. She hated to come late because the head librarian would always fuss if she did so. But this morning she received an urgent phone call from her daughter, and had to talk before heading for the bus. She saw the bus coming and had to rush the last half block to catch it. She made it, but felt a squeezing pain right in the middle of her chest. It was quite uncomfortable, but disappeared about 5 minutes after she sat down. This was the third time she had experienced such a discomfort. She hesitated to call it a pain; it was rather a deep uncomfortable squeezing sensation. The other times she had this sensation were also when she was late and was rushing. She debated seeing her doctor about this problem, but did so after the discomfort occurred a few more times. Her doctor referred her to our office for evaluation. A treadmill exercise, which was predictably abnormal, was strongly positive. Coronary angiography revealed an 80 percent narrowing in the early part of the left anterior descending coronary artery. The area was successfully balloon dilated and after a stent was placed at that site the vessel returned back to normal size. Mrs. F's angina disappeared.

It is fortunate that Mrs. F. decided to see her doctor. She provided a rather classic story of new onset angina pectoris. The pain is usually not severe, but it is often discomfiting. It generally lasts a few minutes to about 10 minutes and is relieved by rest or nitroglycerine taken under the tongue. The typical pain is in the middle of the chest and feels like a squeezing, tightness, or heaviness behind the breastbone. It may be associated with a feeling of breathlessness and in some patients it causes a vague sense of anxiety. The pain may radiate, and be felt in additional places. Sometimes the angina is associated with an aching in the jaw or a feeling of tightness in the throat. Or it may be accompanied by a feeling of tightness or deep aching along the left side of the neck, in the left shoulder, in the left forearm or even in the left wrist. Occasionally the anginal pain will be felt in one of the more distant sites alone and will have no component of chest pain. One of my partners had a patient (to be discussed later) whose anginal pain, a rather deep aching, was felt only in the left thumb with exercise.

No correlation exists between the presence of angina and the severity of the heart disease. Thus, angina may be due to relatively localized coronary artery disease, or may herald severe, extensive disease. That is why it is so important for the doctor to assess the patient's symptoms. Sometimes the pain in the chest will not be due to heart disease at all, but to lower esophageal spasm.

Mr. G.M., a 37-year old accountant, was a committed jogger. He jogged every day, rain or shine, holiday or workday, and felt miserable if he hadn't run his required 3 miles. Lately, his digestion had become rather rotten. He was getting a lot of 'heartburn' for which he was taking Tums and he thought that he should be cutting down on his beer and coffee, but he hated to give up those two strong cups of coffee in the morning that got him going for the day. For the last 3 weeks he had noticed that while running he was developing a feeling of tightness low in the middle of his chest. It was quite unpleasant, and on a couple of occasions he actually stopped running because of it. We found nothing unusual on examination and a treadmill exercise test was quite normal, though Mr. M. complained of the chest squeezing when jogging on the treadmill. Because of his worrisome symptoms, coronary angiography was done and revealed normal coronary arteries. He was referred to a gastroenterologist, who made the diagnosis of an esophageal reflux syndrome and recurrent lower esophageal spasm after certain special studies. The chest discomfort disappeared after the patient improved his diet, eliminated liquor and coffee, and was put on medication to cut down the acid secretions of the stomach.

Though I have detailed this brief history of a real patient, it should be understood that the esophageal origin for an angina type of pain that occurs with such activity as jogging is not common. We must remember that a chest pain brought on by physical exertion or emotional stress requires evaluation by a physician.

Patients with angina pectoris can live for many years. In the days before sophisticated treatments my father lived for at least 12 years, until age 97 years, with angina. He modified his lifestyle and always had nitroglycerine with him, but in general he did quite well. Many effective medications now are available to help the angina patient, though the presence of angina often calls for some modifications in style of life.

Unstable angina pectoris
When angina pectoris changes its characteristics from a predictable and hence stable occurrence, it is termed "unstable." (**Figure 20**). Unstable angina is a serious condition and calls for immediate medical attention and usually hospitalization for study.

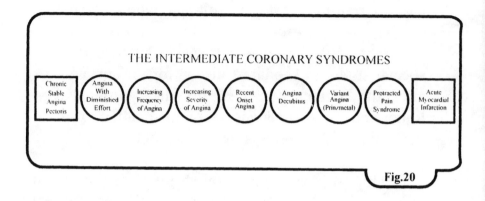

THE INTERMEDIATE CORONARY SYNDROMES

Chronic Stable Angina Pectoris | Angina With Diminished Effort | Increasing Frequency of Angina | Increasing Severity of Angina | Recent Onset Angina | Angina Decubitus | Variant Angina (Prinzmetal) | Protracted Pain Syndrome | Acute Myocardial Infarction

Fig.20

Stable angina pectoris is considered to have become "unstable" when:

- The pain persists in spite of rest or placing nitroglycerine under the tongue.
- The pain occurs with minimal effort, less than previously.
- The pain becomes more frequent than previously.
- The angina occurs at rest or awakens the patient from sleep.

In addition, we consider that the new onset of angina pectoris represents an "unstable" state.

These changes in the nature of a previously stable condition herald a change in the underlying pathology of the coronary arteries and demand medical evaluation. This is, therefore, a time "to worry." Much can be done for such a patient, including medication and, at times, invasive procedures. Thus it is sad to see a person procrastinate and delay medical care.

Mr. R.C., a 67-year old, brilliant physicist, had chronic angina pectoris. He had continued to work, his services being invaluable at his institution. He would get a squeezing pain in the middle of the chest with physical stress, such as walking too fast, or with emotional stress. He would get the pain when he felt exhilarated. He knew his pain was angina pectoris and that it came from heart trouble. Indeed, he had researched the condition before he came to see me. But he adamantly refused diagnostic studies and insisted that he could live with the problem by making adjustments like walking slower and avoiding arguments and stress. Indeed, he moderated his life style and did pretty well, experiencing angina pectoris only about twice weekly. He continued in this more constricted way of life for around eight years, with various medications to decrease the work of the heart muscle and improve its blood supply. He was at work in the laboratory one day when he was seized with a severe pain in the front of the chest, much more severe than usual, that radiated to the left shoulder and down his left arm to the wrist. He felt short of breath. The pain persisted in spite of his taking nitroglycerine tablets under the tongue, and then he felt lightheaded and sweaty. His colleagues called an ambulance and he was taken to our hospital. His condition was stabilized with medications and he became pain free. Diagnostic coronary angiography revealed severe triple vessel disease, but no evidence of a myocardial infarction.

He had coronary bypass surgery a few days later and has been pain free for eight years.

The story of this gentleman illustrates the point made previously, that one can live with angina pectoris for many years. Aside from the issue of longevity and the desirable prevention of a heart attack, quality of life can be markedly enhanced by strategically utilized medical and surgical interventions.

CHAPTER IX

HEART DISEASE |

MANIFESTED BY

PAINS OUTSIDE THE CHEST |

Because pain can be referred from its point of origin, heart disease sometimes manifests with pain outside the chest. The following history of a man treated by one of my partners illustrates the challenge of interpreting referred pain.

Mr. T.T., a 44-year old engineer, was told that his routine electrocardiogram was not normal and he was advised to see a cardiologist. When seen initially, he insisted that he was in good health and that he had absolutely no symptoms related to his heart. The physical examination was completely normal. His weight and blood pressure were normal, and in particular the heart examination was normal. At the time of a treadmill exercise test, during which the electrocardiogram showed marked abnormalities, the patient commented that he was experiencing a severe aching in his left thumb. He noted that such aching had been occurring during the previous 6 months when he exercised or felt rushed, but he had dismissed this symptom as of no significance. Because of the markedly abnormal exercise test and the aching thumb with exercise, Mr. T. was referred for coronary angiography. He proved to have significant coronary artery disease, underwent coronary bypass surgery without event, and his aching thumb with exertion syndrome completely disappeared.

This patient had angina pectoris manifested by pain in the thumb, which is most unusual. However, it is not rare for angina pectoris to manifest itself as a localized pain outside of the chest. The symptom may be aching in the wrist, usually the left, or an aching pain in the left side of the jaw or the left side of the neck or in the throat. The discomfort invariably occurs with exertion or emotional stress. Angina occurring just in the jaw is less rare than thumb pain, but is not common. Patients with this type of discomfort sometimes go to the dentist.

Ms. T.U., an athletic 44-year old post-menopausal high school physical education teacher, was referred to me by her dentist. She had seen him because of recurrent aching in the left lower jaw that occurred after eating and when she felt stressed, and she was convinced that she had a bad tooth. He examined her teeth, obtained x-rays, and could find no evidence of dental decay that would cause her pain. On her insistence, he did some special tests looking for dental trouble, and these tests were also entirely negative. The dentist, a bright and imaginative professional, referred her to our office after he ascertained that the patient's pain not only occurred after eating, but also occurred with emotional stress. The history that I obtained concurred with the dentist's, namely, that with emotional stress the patient was getting left lower jaw pain. The family history included considerable coronary artery disease as well as diabetes. Blood sugars revealed that the patient had early diabetes. A stress echocardiogram was abnormal. Coronary angiography revealed a localized 80 percent narrowing in the left circumflex artery, which the invasive cardiologist dilated and stented. Thereafter Ms. U. had no further jaw pain.

It is surprising, but pain on the left side of the chest in the nipple area is rarely from the heart. However, the rare exceptions demand a high level of suspicion from doctors. Some years ago I had an elderly man with known coronary artery disease in the hospital with pneumonia. During the hospitalization, when he was recovering from the pneumonia, he developed a rather severe pain in the left chest that he insisted was different from the pain of pneumonia. He turned out to be correct; our studies confirmed that he had had an acute myocardial infarction ("heart attack").

Pain in "the pit of the stomach" (the area just below the breastbone; the bottom of the breastbone is where the lowest ribs flare out to the sides) can be due to heart trouble. If a pain in this area comes on with exercise, exertion or emotional stress, consideration should be given to the possibility that it originates from the heart.

Mr. H.Z., a 66-year old, obese jewelry retailer, had been treated by his family doctor for many years for esophageal reflux, heartburn and a duodenal ulcer that had bled on one occasion. The patient lived with regularly occurring pain in the epigastric region ("the pit of the stomach") because of his frequent food indiscretions, alcohol, and coffee. He would treat himself with antacids, in addition to the medication from his doctor to decrease acid secretions from the stomach. On Christmas day, after a surfeit of rich foods and alcohol, Mr. A. developed a severe pain "in the pit of the stomach." The pain became quite intense and was not relieved with antacids and Pepcid. The persistent pain became intolerable and so the patient was taken to our hospital emergency room. An electrocardiogram was markedly abnormal and was consistent with an ongoing acute myocardial infarction ("heart attack"). The patient was immediately taken to the cardiac catheterization laboratory, where coronary angiography revealed significant coronary artery disease and a very tight lesion in the mid left coronary artery. This lesion was balloon dilated and stented, at which time the patient's pain disappeared. Studies later revealed that he had suffered a moderately large myocardial infarction. We explained to Mr. Z. that he would have to modify his lifestyle, lose weight, shift from a wholly sedentary way of life to regular physical activity, and accept treatment of his elevated cholesterol.

As has been stressed, heart disease can manifest through pain in various referred locations without accompanying pain in the middle of the chest. I have emphasized that pain due to heart disease often occurs in the throat, jaw, shoulder, elbow or wrist, and at times in unexpected locations such as the left thumb. The alert physician suspects the significance of these pains because they come on with physical or emotional stress and are relieved by rest. They are not related to particular bodily movements. In the patient presented above, the persistence of the pain in an unusual location for heart pain led to the correct diagnosis and treatment because the nature of the pain and its persistence differed from what the patient usually felt.

Sometimes a change in the location in which chronic angina manifests is a signal of increasing trouble. A change in location of the angina may be a clue to a change in the underlying pathology.

Mrs. R.P., a schoolteacher, 53 years of age, had been experiencing angina on exertion for about two years. Her pain always occurred on the left side of the jaw and in the throat and was precipitated by strenuous activity such as hurrying up two flights of stairs with groceries or rushing for an appointment. On her medical regimen she averaged about one episode a week, knew that she had angina pectoris, and used nitroglycerine under the tongue with relief of discomfort. Indeed, she had learned to use the nitroglycerine prophylactically before being faced with predictable angina-producing situations. In the week preceding her visit to our offices the angina that she experienced occurred as usual and she felt it in the left side of the jaw and the throat, but now she also experienced an uncomfortable squeezing sensation in the middle of her chest. This latter pain persisted longer than the jaw pain and worried her a good deal. We hospitalized her and studies revealed a very tight narrowing in a major coronary artery that was balloon dilated and stented. Much to everyone's delight, her jaw and throat pain disappeared, as did the pain in the middle of the chest.

This patient illustrates something that has been stressed before when we discussed unstable angina pectoris, but it merits emphasizing again. A change in the pattern of pain is often an important clue that the underlying pathology has changed and that further evaluation is necessary.

CHAPTER X

CHEST PAINS
THE COMPANY THEY KEEP &

The symptoms and signs that accompany chest pain or pain in one of the referred sites for heart disease are very important in assessing the significance of the pain. These associated symptoms, as well as the circumstances under which they occur, often lead the clinician to the correct diagnosis. Some of the symptoms and signs have already been discussed; for example, we discussed the classic example of the jogger who gets a pressing pain in the front of the chest that turns out to be due to reflux (regurgitation) into the esophagus from the stomach. The correct diagnosis was made after considering all the clinical factors and then doing studies to rule out heart disease. The fact that a patient drinks strong coffee, likes martinis and eats spicy foods is important diagnostically. The jogger had a perfectly normal treadmill exercise test, with normal blood pressure responses, which also was significant. He was on the treadmill for 12 minutes, a finding consistent with excellent physical condition and not suggestive of heart disease.

Sometimes the nature of the physical activity that brings on a pain leads to the correct diagnosis.

Mr. J.S., a 35-year old, machine tool operator, complained of a deep aching left shoulder pain on exertion. When asked for examples of what brought on the shoulder pain, he described it as occurring when sweeping the floor where he worked or when working in his yard. On questioning it turned out that he never had the pain when he was rushed or when out jogging his usual three times a week. With a treadmill exercise test the patient's performance was athletic, his heart rate and blood pressure responses were normal, as were the electrocardiograms. There was no evidence of heart disease. He was referred to an orthopedist, who made the diagnosis of a tendintis involving the left shoulder. Clearly, it was not the level of physical exertion that brought on this man's pain, but rather the fact that he engaged in certain physical movements.

I once saw a lady, 55 years of age, who complained of pain in the left shoulder and was very concerned that it was pain from her heart. She was left-handed, and generally her pain was precipitated by reaching up, especially reaching up to get things off her higher kitchen shelves. She also had shoulder discomfort when bowling. Careful questioning revealed that she would also get similar pain in the right shoulder with certain movements. It was obvious that her pain had nothing to do with the heart. She was understandably worried about her heart because her mother had died when she was in her late 50s from heart disease.

In some instances a chest pain is associated with a life circumstance or event that likely explains its origin.

Mrs. K.K., a 60-year old housewife and social worker, presented herself with the complaint of a persistent load, a feeling of heaviness, in the front of the chest. The heaviness would come and go, but when present would persist for hours at a time. Her discomfort had started about three weeks previously. The usual medical questions suggested no pathology and, in fact, there was much to suggest that Mrs. K's cardiac health was excellent. During the physical examination, when asked how life was treating her these days, she started to cry. The physical examination was completely normal, as was an electrocardiogram, but when asked about her tears Mrs. K told me that about one month previously her daughter had given birth to a child with Down's syndrome, and the patient was terribly depressed and anxious for her daughter. The heaviness on her chest was the result of grief, not an unusual symptom with great emotional stress or overwhelming events such as the death of a loved one.

Mrs. K. provides an example of grief causing a particular type of chest pain. Even though grief and depression might explain the pain, the doctor must take care to rule out heart disease. The reader should remember that a sensation of heaviness in the chest is defined as a type of "pain" by doctors. In this instance the patient felt better after talking about her misery with me. I explained to her that she and her daughter would be well advised to obtain psychological counseling.

The important lesson of these examples is that pain from the heart usually is related to physical or emotional stress that throws a load on the heart and, as I have reiterated so often, not all chest pains are due to heart trouble.

Chest pains and cardiac abnormalities may occur as part of systemic disease that includes many body symptoms. Persons suffering a stroke will often have abnormal heart findings. Diabetes mellitus is a major risk factor for atherosclerosis of the coronary and peripheral arteries. Neurological disorders may co-exist with heart problems as, for example in certain congenital heart conditions. Rheumatoid arthritis can be associated with heart valve disease. The condition of prolapse of the mitral valve is sometimes associated with complaints of chest pain and palpitations due to premature heart beats. Abnormal function of the thyroid gland is associated with heart symptoms, and disturbances of the body electrolytes can be associated with abnormal heart rhythms. For correct diagnosis and treatment the skilled cardiologist must have a reasonable knowledge of all body systems.

CHAPTER XI

REVIEWING
WHEN TO WORRY & WHEN TO RELAX

Reading this book can provide information and help you assess chest pain, but it can provide no guarantees of infallible judgement thereafter. A reasonable concern, tempered with a sensible knowledge about the organs of the chest, is the best approach to good health for most of us. My hope is that this book will encourage the reader to that state of awareness. Do keep in mind that it is not a good idea to be cavalier with chest pain of unknown origin. Experienced doctors know that!

It is true that the main concern for individuals with chest pain is the heart. But protracted chest pain of any kind merits attention. It may prove to have nothing to do with the heart or lungs, but one is entitled to a diagnosis and relief from pain even if it is not serious or life threatening. Indeed, any kind of protracted pain, including that not in the chest, calls for medical evaluation.

Severe pain in the front of the chest, with or without radiation to the arm, neck or jaw, merits immediate action, and that includes dialing 911 and getting to a hospital emergency room. Don't waste time trying to reach your doctor under such circumstances; the emergency room physicians can contact him. Don't procrastinate. If the pain turns out to be esophageal spasm or indigestion or muscular rather than heart trouble, just be relieved, not embarrassed or guilty. You paid your taxes and your health insurance premiums and are entitled to the medical care you got. If someone close to you, a relative or friend, suffers such a pain and wants to wait a while - "Let's see if the pain will go away in an hour or so while we try to reach the doctor" - don't acquiesce! Insist on acting appropriately and call 911. Medical care has so much to offer if a heart injury is occurring that it is a serious mistake to procrastinate. Procrastination may have lasting consequences in resulting in permanent heart damage and even death. Recurrent chest pain of the kinds we have covered, or pain in one of the areas of referral that have been discussed, especially when brought on by physical or emotional stress should send one to the doctor. Pain brought on by exertion after eating is a must to see the doctor. Keep in mind that the pain does not have to be severe, that it can be a mild pressure or squeezing or heaviness, and nevertheless calls for attention. If the discomfort is in the center of the chest, behind the breastbone, it deserves evaluation. At times the discomfort may not be in the center of the chest, and may be in the shoulder or jaw or arm. If it is related to emotional or physical stress, it should not be dismissed.

We have learned that some chest pains occur with acute emotional stress, such as having an argument with a spouse or getting very angry with a co-worker. Severe emotional stress can precipitate a myocardial infarction in a susceptible person. Emotional stress is also a potent stimulant for anginal pain. Pain brought on by acute emotional stress merits the same kind of attention as pain precipitated by physical work. The death of a loved one, or the onset of a chronic disease in oneself or a loved one, represents a sustained emotional stress, which can be experienced as a persistent and recurrent heaviness in the chest. This symptom often goes with grief and depression. Wisdom dictates that the person with a symptom as chest heaviness related to sustained emotional stress see a doctor, particularly when there are accompanying symptoms such as palpitations, weakness or faintness. Such emotional stress does not rule out concurrent heart trouble.

Recurrent "heartburn" after imbibing coffee or alcohol, or after eating spicy food, is usually from esophageal reflux. On occasion, burning pain in the middle of the chest can be from the heart. Even if symptoms are indicative of heartburn rather than heart trouble, "heartburn" can be a chronic misery and can be associated with esophageal injury. There is good treatment available. So why suffer? Get it checked out by your physician.

Some persons have never had a chest pain. Let us assume that such an individual gets a chest pain for the first time, never having had such a pain before. It should not be ignored, and certainly if it recurs it should be checked.

Dr. S.T. was a 52-year old dentist who was a committed jogger. He jogged at least two miles every day, rain or shine, hail or sleet, and had been doing this for about 25 years. He always felt better when he got done with his morning run. About two months before he came to be examined he had noted that when he started to run he developed a peculiar, mild tightness in the middle of his chest. But as he continued to run, within about three minutes the tightness disappeared and he had no further discomfort. In view of this scenario he concluded that this minimal pain was of no consequence. But soon he noted that the chest discomfort occurred when he was late for an appointment and was rushing to get there. That, and the death of a close friend from a heart attack, convinced him to see a doctor. He proved to have significant coronary artery disease on coronary angiography. He resumed his jogging without discomfort after he had angioplasty and stenting of two vessels. He also was started on medications to prevent progression of his disease.

This patient had a variety of anginal pattern in which the pain goes away even though the exercise is continued. As the case history demonstrates, the pain still merits evaluation.

There are chest pains that are so clearly musculoskeletal in origin that consultation with a cardiologist is unnecessary. For example, pain in the neck, shoulder and the upper right side of the chest that first occurs after a peculiar swing when serving during a game of tennis and that recurs with certain arm and head movements is surely musculoskeletal in origin. Tightness across the top of the chest the day after experiencing a whiplash injury to the neck is very likely muscular in origin. A painful elbow that feels warm and hurts on pressure is clearly not from the heart.

Table 3A-B lists some pertinent points about "when to worry," but do keep in mind that it is important to err on the side of caution. When in doubt see a physician. And has been emphasized before, a change in the quality or pattern of a chest pain calls for evaluation by a physician.

Sometimes it is impossible for a person to describe his or her situation, and yet the person knows that something is not right. Maybe the pain aspect of the situation is very minimal, but there are other symptoms, like fatigue, awareness of heart irregularities, shortness of breath with only moderate exertion, lightheadedness or faintness with activity, and so on. Under such circumstances, a person should not hesitate "to worry" and to consult a physician. After all, many heart problems of a serious nature do not manifest pain at all, or the pain is a minor aspect of the person's discomfort. Though we are dealing with chest pain, it should be emphasized that heart trouble is often signaled by shortness of breath or the onset of unusual fatigue. Dizziness, faintness, fainting, heart racing and palpitations can indicate significant heart problems. Being a smart patient prepared to take advantage of the remarkable advances in medicine involves not only some knowledge, but also a reasonable awareness of one's body and a commitment to taking good care oneself.

CHAPTER XII

A REVIEW|
———————— OF WHAT TO DO WHEN
CHEST PAIN COMES |

A "not to worry" chest pain, such as those noted in **Table 3A-B**, is not cause for alarm or haste in seeing a doctor. However, even a "not to worry" pain in the chest that is persistent or nagging and recurrent merits evaluation by a physician on a non-urgent basis.

Severe pain, particularly when it occurs in the middle of the chest, with or without radiation of the pain represents a time to worry and to act. Even if the pain eases up, it should be evaluated. Less severe pain that persists, whether or not it radiates to the neck or arm or one of the other less common sites we have discussed, particularly if accompanied by symptoms such as weakness or faintness or palpitations, also merits immediate action. A person's understandable anxiety in such a situation should not lead to being incapacitated to act properly. Be smart about your body! Even when in doubt, getting to a hospital emergency room as soon as possible is the proper response. You or a close by person should dial 911 without hesitation. If you are in a rural area, have someone take you straight to the closest hospital. Do not monkey around with trying to reach the doctor by phone or worrying about what your managed care plan will say or do. Let the doctors decide whether the pain is or is not a serious one. And if it turns out to be a false alarm - wonderful!

The heart usually signals being in trouble with chest pain in the front of the chest or in the areas that have been discussed as frequent sites of pain radiation. Pain originating from the heart usually is brought on by physical exertion or emotional stress. But this is not always true. Acute heart episodes, like a myocardial infarction ("heart attack"), can occur while one is comfortably seated and relaxed. And one of the characteristics of unstable angina is that it may occur at rest. As emphasized, heart trouble can be signaled by shortness of breath, unusual weakness, palpitations, faintness and other general symptoms with or without chest pain. A severe pain on the side of the chest that is persistent, perhaps worse with breathing in, with or without other symptoms like chills or fever, merits attention by a physician. Examples of conditions that can cause this kind of pain include a blood clot to the lung, pleurisy and pneumonia.

The tools that doctors have to differentiate serious from benign chest pain are sophisticated and effective (see the next chapter). Most of the tests we order are not

PAINS MERITING WORRY AND ACTION

- Severe pain in the middle of the chest, a squeezing, pressure or heaviness, often associated with a feeling of shortness of breath.
- Deep, aching pain, squeezing, constricting, a pressure or heaviness, in the middle of the chest, at the base of the neck, left side of neck, throat, shoulder, left arm, left wrist or hand brought on by rushing, physical or emotional stress, particularly after a meal, and relieved with rest.
- Pain in the middle of the chest, not necessarily severe, a tightness, constriction, squeezing or heaviness occurring at rest and persisting.
- Pain in the middle of the chest, neck, throat, shoulder, or left arm awakening one at night and persisting.
- Mild pain or discomfort in the middle of the chest or in one of the other heart pain referral sites associated with marked weakness, lightheadedness, rapid or irregular pulse.
- An unexplained discomfiting pain, persistent or recurrent, merits medical evaluation, irrespective of where it is.
- Chest pain aggravated by inspiration. Sudden onset, sometimes with cough, sometimes with coughing pinkish sputum.

Table-3A

associated with any significant degree of discomfort, the worst discomfort usually being drawing of blood, the establishing of an intravenous line and the necessity for the patient to lie still while various kinds of "pictures"

121

PAINS AND SENSATIONS RARELY MERITING WORRY

- Sharp, shooting pains.
- Sharp transitory pains on the left side of the chest.
- "Heartburn" after eating spicy foods or after alcohol or coffee consumption relieved with milk or an antacid. May merit medical evaluation for esophagus or stomach problems.
- Aching pains in arms or shoulders brought on by certain movements, but not related to running or rushing or emotional stress.
- Aching chest pains that are recurrent, often associated with tenderness on pressure, last for hours and are eased by heat, aspirin or acetaminophen.
- Numbness or tingling in hands or fingers after sleeping on the side that disappears soon after awakening and getting out of bed.

Table-3B

are taken. Even when coronary angiography becomes necessary, it being the most invasive diagnostic procedure, it is generally done with great safety and remarkably little discomfort to the patient. Many of my patients report having slept through the procedure. It is impossible for me to list every kind of chest discomfort that should get a patient to the hospital, but the important message is that if in doubt, go to the hospital emergency room without delay.

CHAPTER XIII

THE PREVENTION

OF CORONARY ARTERY DISEASE

&

THE PREVENTION OF ITS PROGRESSION

The prevention of heart disease merits our committed attention. The prevention of coronary atherosclerosis ("hardening of the arteries") and the avoidance of its progression to angina or heart attack is well worth the effort entailed. The lifestyle adjustments to prevent coronary artery disease and strokes should undoubtedly start at an early age, when persons are in their 20s or even younger. It is likely that in the future doctors will be able to look at the genetic structure of every patient and will determine which ones are particularly susceptible to certain diseases, such as coronary atherosclerosis. Indeed, gene therapy may be able to alter such susceptibilities. However, until that day comes the reality in our society is that prevention is usually "secondary." That is, "prevention" is directed at avoiding progression of disease in those patients who already have evidence of coronary atherosclerosis.

Certainly if a person has ever had a heart muscle injury the avoidance of future trouble is critically important. That is unequivocally true for those patients who have had coronary angioplasty or coronary bypass surgery, where it is desirable to stabilize whatever disease is present and to block its progression.

If one has never had heart trouble, it is sensible to do the things that we know can markedly decrease one's chance of having trouble in the future. Patients with diabetes mellitus are highly at risk and should be especially disciplined in following the right paths to forestall coronary heart disease. I know one diabetes specialist who routinely sends his patients over the age of 35 years for a cardiac evaluation. Persons with a significant family history of coronary heart disease should also give particular attention to the risk factors for this disease. The following simple rules are applicable for every adult, even those without elevated risk of heart disease:

- See to it that your blood pressure is normal, taking medication if necessary.
- Do not smoke cigarettes, a pipe or cigars. Whenever possible, avoid secondary exposure to tobacco smoke.
- Watch your diet. Keep your weight down. Avoid foods with high fat high cholesterol content.
- If you have diabetes, commit yourself to a proper diet and excellent blood sugar control. There is increasing evidence that a low carbohydrate, relatively high protein diet is desirable for diabetics. Consult your physician

about your diet.

- Maintain a program of regular physical activity. Remember the motto: "Walkers live longer!"
- Younger patients with significant family histories of coronary heart disease should have their blood lipids checked. Checking the blood homocysteine level, a factor predisposing to atherosclerosis, is also desirable.

There is a vast body of evidence showing that an abnormally elevated blood cholesterol is undesirable and predisposes to coronary atheroscerosis. The total fasting cholesterol should be below 200 mg/DL. The LDL (low density lipoprotein) is the undesirable fraction and the generally accepted recommendation for patients with coronary artery disease is to keep it below 100 mg/DL. There are physicians who try to get their patients to achieve even lower levels. The HDL (the high density lipoprotein) is the desirable fraction, and it is ideally above 50 mg/DL. Some physicians pay a good deal of attention to the total cholesterol/HDL ratio, with under 3.0 being desirable for patients with coronary artery disease. Many physicians are paying more attention to the blood triglyceride levels. This fat in the blood must be measured with the patient in the fasting state.

A Mediterranean diet, with a high intake of fruits and vegetables is desirable. Modest amounts of wine are usually acceptable. Have your cholesterol, its undesirable fraction (LDL) and good cholesterol fraction (HDL) in as close to the ideal range as possible.

In some instances medication to help will be necessary and should be used.

A normal cholesterol level is unquestionably desirable, but it is by no means the total answer to preventing arterial disease. Good blood pressure control has great dividends, including fewer undesirable cardiac events and far fewer strokes. Moreover, good blood pressure control helps prevent heart failure, kidney and eye damage. Accurate blood pressure measuring devices have become quite inexpensive and patients can easily check blood pressures at home on a routine suggested by the physician. Such blood pressure determinations are of considerable value to the physician in helping control the blood pressure. Indeed, I rely heavily on such blood pressure information from patients, it in many ways being more helpful than occasional blood pressures taken in the doctor's office.

Exercise is important, and becomes more important as we get older. Muscles need work to retain function and strength. I often recommend that patients exercise 15 minutes every day, using a treadmill, a bicycle and modest sized weights. Calisthenics to maintain muscle range of motion are helpful. Many people like water exercises, and they are excellent. Walking, making a bed, vacuuming the rugs, going grocery shopping, walking up the stairs, gardening - all such activities involve muscle exercise and are useful. The couch-potato mentality that drives the car to get the newspaper one block away is to be avoided.

There is good evidence that persons following the relatively simple desirable lifestyle habits that are listed can significantly increase their quality of life as well as their life expectancy. It doesn't take genius to understand that the prevention of heart trouble, peripheral arterial disease and strokes is very important in enhancing the quality of one's life.

CHAPTER XIV

THE STUDIES & TEST |
—————————— IN DIAGNOSIS OF
HEART DISEASE |

- *The medical history:*
    A careful history is critical to the diagnosis of chest pain. Sometimes obtaining a complete history is not possible when a patient is having severe pain, and under such circumstances emergency medical intervention takes precedent. However, when the pain or discomfort is eased or relieved, then a more detailed history is obtained whenever possible. The history usually provides direction concerning which tests should be ordered to clarify the diagnosis. It takes the doctor time and concentration to get a complete history, and an informed patient who can describe their kind and site of discomfort is of great help. I like to take a complete history on every new patient I see, whether referred by another physician or self-referred.

- *The physical examination:*

In an emergency, the physical examination will usually be directed by the history and the nature and location of the pain. Particular attention will generally be paid to examining the heart, lungs, abdomen and extremities. Depending on the circumstances, a more detailed physical examination will provide more information. When possible, I like to do a relatively complete examination in a patient with chest pain, because examination of other organs may offer important clues to the correct diagnosis. For example, the absence of arterial pulses in the feet is important evidence of probable generalized atherosclerosis.

- *The electrocardiogram:*

The electrocardiogram is the first line of testing for patients who have chest pain or pain elsewhere that presents in such a way as to suggest the possibility of heart trouble. It is a painless test that registers the electrical currents in the heart by putting pickup leads on various parts of the surface of the body. It is a superb tool for revealing heart muscle injury. Often serial electrocardiograms taken over time intervals of varying length will give valuable information. The patient with chest pain admitted to a hospital emergency room is always hooked up to a continuous electrocardiographic monitor, it being the ideal method to observe the heart rhythm. The well trained cardiologist is also an expert electrocardiographer.

- *Chest x-rays*

Chest x-rays reveal the heart size and shape and

help clarify the status of the lungs. The heart may be enlarged or have an atypical shape, as in certain kinds of rheumatic heart disease. The aorta (the large vessel arising from the left ventricle) can be visualized and its size determined in order to alert us to abnormalities. For example, an aneurysm of the aorta may be visible. Pneumonia and other lung problems, such as an embolus of a blood clot to the lung, can often be diagnosed with a chest x-ray. More recently there has been an increase in lung tuberculosis, and of course the chest x-ray is important in making this diagnosis. Years ago fluoroscopy of the heart and lungs was a common office test, but it has been abandoned because of excessive radiation exposure to the patient. To a great extent, echocardiography has supplanted the chest x-ray as a superior method of studying the heart, but the chest x-rays remain very important in the evaluation for lung disease. Sometimes findings in the lungs seen on chest x-rays will help clarify a patient's heart condition.

- *Blood studies, including heart enzymes*

A complete blood count is often obtained to rule out such conditions as anemia or infection. Electrolytes, such as potassium and sodium, are usually checked, and are important in understanding certain abnormal heart rhythms. Blood tests assessing kidney function are important in evaluating heart conditions. Thyroid function tests are often desirable. The blood sugar is routinely checked, because it is particularly important to know if the patient has diabetes. In certain instances blood homocysteine levels are obtained. Other blood studies can be done depending on the diagnoses being considered. For example, a blood calcium level may reveal overactivity of parathyroid glands, which can affect the heart.

Various enzymes (CPK and troponins I and T) are released from the injured heart, almost always from the left ventricle muscle when it is not receiving enough blood and oxygen. It usually takes some time after injury before the blood drawn from a vein shows significant levels of these enzymes, but when they become elevated it is important evidence that a portion of the heart muscle has been injured. The degree of elevation of these enzymes provides evidence for the extent of the heart muscle damage. The troponin levels have markedly influenced our approach to the patient with chest pain, becoming extremely important in diagnosis.

- *Lipid profile*
  The determination of blood triglycerides, cholesterol and its fractions (HDL and LDL) is mandatory in studying a patient with cardiovascular disease. It is necessary to obtain the levels of high density lipoproteins (HDL) and low density lipoproteins (LDL). They are of little value in acute emergency conditions, but are very desirable to define a program for the care of these patients. Blood triglycerides must be obtained with the patient in a fasting state.

- *C reactive protein and other blood tests*
  C reactive protein and other blood tests, including the sedimentation rate, provide evidence of

inflammation and infection. Such tests recently have been cited as evidence that infection may play a role in causing coronary atherosclerosis. We know that inflammation is a part of the atherosclerotic plaque, but the question of infection by a virus or bacteria remains an area of hypothesis and experiment, and much more data are needed. The sedimentation rate is of help in following patients with rheumatic fever, pericarditis and bacterial endocarditis (infection of heart valve). Tests for inflammation in the body likely will become of increasing value in diagnosing heart disease.

- *Treadmill exercise ("stress") test:*

The treadmill exercise test is valuable in the diagnosis of chest pain, but it has to be used with care. It is not used in the presence of an acute heart muscle injury, but is often helpful in clarifying a chest pain when the resting electrocardiogram is basically normal. At some institutions a bicycle is used in the stress test. Whether using treadmill or bicycle, the exercise test provides information about the blood pressure, heart rate and physical endurance, as well as demonstrating electrocardiographic changes. Certain changes in the electrocardiograms, associated with exercise, indicate that an area of heart muscle is not receiving enough blood for that level of exertion. At some medical institutions the treadmill exercise test is performed in or near the emergency room to help physicians determine which patients presenting with chest pain should be hospitalized and which ones can be allowed to go home.

- *The fast CT scan for coronary artery calcium:*

If one pays heed to the radio and newspaper advertisements one has to conclude that this is the screening test that every adult should have and that it provides information that leads to the solution of all heart problems. In fact the test does have value on occasion when it is used and interpreted appropriately. It is true that calcium in the coronary arteries reflects the presence of atherosclerosis, but this test, which shows the amount of calcium in the coronary arteries, gives no information about the functional state of the coronary arteries and the heart. In other words, it does not tell us how much blood is flowing through the coronary arteries to the heart muscle, and that is the critical information. I order this test from time to time, particularly in a younger person without symptoms who has a worrisome family history for coronary artery disease.

- *Echocardiography*

Echocardiography, in which certain kinds of sounds are bounced off the heart structures, provides remarkably clear and accurate images. This technique has become extremely sophisticated and helpful and modern systems allow for miraculous clarity in imaging the heart's contours and its structures. And the engineers keep making it better. With echocardiography, the valves of the heart can be seen, the origins of the great vessels can be visualized, a chamber size and wall thickness can be measured, and the function of the four chambers can be assessed. Injured heart muscle does not move normally and this phenomenon is demonstrated. The echo is an extremely valuable test for almost all kinds of heart trouble, as well as for studying the patient with chest pain. It is also valuable in following the course of cardiac problems. In some cases a small pickup device is passed down the esophagus to the level of the heart to get particularly good images of certain heart structures. This procedure is somewhat uncomfortable for the patient for a relatively short period of time, but often it provides critical information and becomes worth the temporary discomfort.

It is now, appropriately, routine that every patient with a significant cardiac history have an echocardiographic study. The value of the test is remarkable, but as with all such studies, the skill and commitment of the technician who administers the test and the physician who reviews the pictures is important.

● *Stress echocardiography*
Stress echocardiography utilizes this technique to assess the function of the left ventricle immediately after exercise, as well as at rest. Initially the heart is examined by echocardiography with the patient at rest. The patient then is exercised on a treadmill or stationary bicycle to near maximum capacity or until symptoms occur, at which point the exercise is stopped and the heart is re-examined. Much information about heart function can be obtained with this test, with particular interest being centered on the wall motion of the left ventricle, the major heart chamber pumping blood to the body. Certain kinds of abnormal wall motion indicate that the heart muscle is deprived of sufficient blood.

This test is valuable in assessing patients for surgery, and is also valuable in studying patients after coronary artery bypass surgery.

- *Stress echocardiography with dobutamine or adenosine*
  This procedure is used when the patient is unable to exercise adequately on a treadmill, as for example a patient with disabling knee or hip pain. These drugs given by vein in gradually increasing dosage simulate exercise in its effect on the heart. Echocardiography is performed before, during and after the administration of the agent.

- *Radioisotope imaging*
  Certain kinds of imaging can be used to tell how much blood each of the ventricles is pumping out per unit time, a measure known as the "ejection fraction." This information is valuable, and can be obtained with essentially no discomfort to the patient. A significantly injured ventricle is unable to pump a normal volume of blood. In most institutions an ejection fraction over 50 percent is considered normal. Trained athletes may have markedly increased ejection fractions.

- *Stress dual isotope study*
  With this highly sophisticated technique the blood flow to the ventricular muscle (the myocardium) is determined at rest and at the peak of exercise. A mismatch between the flow patterns, for example when flow to a portion of the left ventricle is decreased during exercise but becomes normal at rest, flags an area of the heart muscle that is not getting enough blood with

exercise. One can often determine what part of the heart muscle is receiving insufficient blood by the pattern of the images that are created. In addition, the newer equipment also provides valuable information about how the left ventricle is contracting. For patients who cannot exercise on a treadmill, adenosine may be administered in the vein to increase the work of the heart and thus to assess the coronary blood flow at rest and at the equivalent of exercise.

- *PET scanning*

   This superb technique, which requires highly expensive equipment and the preparation of fresh radioactive isotopes, gives information about the metabolism of the heart muscle under varying circumstances. It remains an experimental tool and is available at only a few institutions in the United States, but offers information that can be valuable in the assessment of chest pain.

- *Magnetic Resonance Imaging*

   MRI already has a valuable role in the assessment of valvular and congenital heart disease. In addition, areas of heart muscle injury can be visualized. MRI holds great promise for the visualization of the normal and abnormal coronary arteries. The technique has been perfected to the point where the initial portions of the coronary arteries are quite well visualized. In the future this technique will become increasingly important in assessing coronary heart disease and chest pain syndromes.

- *Heart catheterization and coronary angiography*

This diagnostic technique, still the gold standard for defining the status of the coronary arteries, has become remarkably sophisticated and is done with great safety in skilled hands. The equipment is superb, the patient is relatively comfortable during the study, and the diagnostic part of the test to view the coronary arteries generally goes very smoothly and lasts less than one hour. During this time the patient lies comfortably on a table, and the doctor moves the equipment depending on the views of the heart that he wants to obtain. Usually the most uncomfortable part of the test is having a local anesthetic injected into the area of the right groin, and a mild sedative is often given before the procedure. The coronary arteries are visualized by injecting small amounts of contrast material (dye) into their openings at the base of the aorta. On rare occasion when a patient is allergic to the contrast material, special preparations with anti-allergic agents can prevent any adverse reactions. Sometimes more extensive diagnostic studies are indicated, with the measurement of pressures and flow in the various chambers. Such studies take longer, but rarely cause the patient any additional discomfort.

Coronary angiography done by skilled so-called "invasive" cardiologists has become so sophisticated that physicians often move from diagnosis directly to treatment, with angioplasty and stenting of significant coronary artery stenoses.

- *24-hour electrocardiographic monitoring (Holter monitoring)*

This diagnostic technique records the heart rhythm over the course of 24 or 48 hours, thus providing valuable information about the heart rhythm under varying life situations, including sleep. On occasion, this technique also provides information on the failure of adequate blood supply to a portion of the heart muscle. It is often called "Holter monitoring" - after Dr. Holter who devised it. It involves the patient being "hooked up" with special electrocardiographic electrodes and carrying a small recording device. It is all quite painless, but one cannot bathe while wearing this costly equipment.

- *24-hour blood pressure monitoring*

This valuable procedure, which consists of repeated blood pressures being recorded over a 24-hour period, usually remains classified as a research tool. At the present time its use is not covered by any of the insurance companies, though Medicare does provide reimbursement under certain conditions. We have the equipment in our office, where we have used it primarily in research studies. When utilized it can provide important information about a patient's blood pressure variations during various life circumstances and sleep, and it is such equipment that has given us information about normal blood pressures during sleep and during the different parts of the day.

- *Other tests*

Many additional tests are available to the

physician and have an occasional role in the diagnosis of chest pain. I mention them here, but will not go into detail concerning them. They include psychological testing, esophageal studies, upper gastrointestinal and gall bladder x-rays, x-rays of the cervical and dorsal spine, pulmonary function testing, finger oximetry at rest and after exercise, and spiral CT scan. I am sure that additional tests will be forthcoming considering the remarkable technological advances in our society.

Do keep in mind what I said at the beginning of this chapter: the properly done history and physical examination are the procedures that provide the information leading to appropriate testing. Each of the tests has value under certain clinical circumstances. The patient admitted with the clinical picture of an acute myocardial infarction ("heart attack") merits an electrocardiogram, blood tests and transfer to the catheterization laboratory for coronary angiography and appropriate treatment. If one is at an institution without a catheterization laboratory, treatment with clot-dissolving medications is indicated. On the other hand, a young person with sharp stabbing pains under the left breast requires reassurance, perhaps after getting an electrocardiogram and an echocardiographic study. The skill of the experienced physician includes knowing what tests to utilize to provide the safest course and best information to serve the patient.

The author is indebted to the many patients who have provided the experience leading to this book. Indeed, it has been suggestions from patients that led to writing it.